Praise for *Love More Now*

"Gigi Langer has hit another home run. *Love More Now* is a kind, gentle guide to her readers on how to improve their lives by opening their hearts to all those souls who have wandered their way. Through honest and very intimate self-disclosure, Gigi shows how her own life has changed by daring to face her past, and have a kinder, more loving present. The real beauty of this book is the clear, loving direction as she explains how you too can change your present."

—**Karen Casey, PhD**, Bestselling Author of *Each Day A New Beginning: Daily Meditations for Women* (Alcoholism recovery; 40th anniversary edition)

"Gigi Langer lays out a framework for change that is insightful and useful, without being prescriptive or overbearing. Her suggestions allow leeway for differing beliefs and experiences, empowering readers to make adaptations that fit their perspectives. The book includes a look at Twelve-Step practices and explains the intent of each step, inviting readers to consider how they might use these and other tools."

—**Jean McCarthy**, Author of *UnPickled: Prepare to be Alcohol-Free*, Producer/Host of *The Bubble Hour* Podcast

"I absolutely LOVE this book, and I see it flying off the shelves. The reader can easily follow the flow because Gigi did such a beautiful job of clarifying the ideas and tools presented."

—**Harriet Hunter**, Author of *Miracles of Recovery: Collector's Edition*

"Langer has penned a real gem for anyone who wants to journey within and shake off the shackles that kept your heart closed. She offers practical examples and exercises to help reawaken your authentic self and embrace all the good life holds for you."

—**Lisa Boucher**, Award-Winning Author of *Raising the Bottom* and *Pray. Trust. Ride: Lessons on Surrender from a Cowgirl and a King*

"Very easy read and thoughtful questions. Perfect for group study in recovery step-work."

—**Angie Cosma**

"Gigi Langer has created a dynamic, interactive book that combines her personal and professional experiences with research and practice. *Love More Now* invites the reader to examine the concept of open-hearted living, analyze what closes one's heart, explore strategies to discover one's true self, and navigate and embrace relationships. The book is punctuated with scenarios, anecdotes, examples, and stories to illustrate ways to embrace life's challenges with open-hearted wisdom. The chapters present a treasure trove of resources to inspire change and growth for anyone who is ready to embark upon a journey to *Love More Now*!"

—**Dr. Pam Robbins**, Author and Celebrated International Public Speaker

"This book is educational, enlightening, and hopeful. It explains how to open up the channel to the true self, even when it's been closed off. I love how we get to 'hold hands while crossing the street of life.' I got a lot out of the sections on being highly sensitive, whispered lies, and the four Rs (Refrain, Reflect, Release, Respond)."

—**Denise McDougal**, Producer/Host of the Recovery Podcast, *Beyond Our Wildest Dreams*

"I highly recommend this inspiring book for anyone who wants a more balanced and heart-centered life. Gigi has written a clear guide with many scenarios, methods, and tools that show how to create positive change and embrace the power of one's true self. Important wisdom from a variety of sources, including Twelve-Step principles and mindfulness, show how forgiveness, joy, and resilience are possible when we learn to open our hearts."

—**Ann Greaver**, Certified Grief Counselor

"I so admire Gigi's honesty and vulnerability in sharing her experiences. It puts so much power and credibility behind what she is writing. This book is so packed with wisdom—and at the same time so practical—with great ways to apply the ideas."

—**Annabelle Nesbit**, Interfaith Minister

"For all who doubt that they are lovable; for all who have trouble seeing the love in their spouse, children, friends, and co-workers, *please pick up this wonderful book.* It will soothe your hearts. Thank you, Gigi, for a further look inside to find the woman my Creator always knew I was."

—**Rev. Barbara Brownyard**, Interfaith, Interspiritual Minister

Love More Now

Facing Life's Challenges with an Open Heart

Love More Now

Gigi Langer, PhD

Possum Hill Press, 488 Veranda Way, Naples, FL 34104

Cover Design and Typography: Susi Clark, *www.CreativeBlueprintDesign.com*
Editors: Teresa Spencer, *terieber@sbcglobal.net* and
Anita LeBlanc, The Write Word, *thewriteword@sbcglobal.net*
Proofreader: Carly Catt, Catt Editing, LLC, *carly@cattediting.com*

First printing 2023

Manufactured in the United States of America

Cataloging-in-Publication Data is available from the Library of Congress.

ISBN: 978-0-9991220-5-1 (Paperback)
ISBN: 978-0-9991220-6-8 (E-Book)

To order, or to learn more, please visit the author's website at www.gigilanger.com. Facebook Gigi Langer Author; Twitter @gigi_langer; Instagram @gigilangerworrylessnow; YouTube @gigilangerphd-worrylessnow4478

All names of friends and family in the stories herein have been changed to protect their anonymity.

Contents

Acknowledgments

A very special thank-you goes to my husband, Peter, my rock and greatest champion. I couldn't have done it without your patience and love…and all those snacks served to me as I was typing away!

I also offer deep gratitude to my circle of friends who support my growth and dreams: Sue Ahrenhold, Ellie Allwein, Liz Audette, Gloria Brooks, Lorilyn Bryan, Ginny Chism, Dawn Champanois, Anna Devlin, Sue DuPree, Cathy Freeman, Eileen Grady, Desiree Haley, Mary Cay Johns, Bethann Jorgenson, Betsy Kirchen, Angelique Lange, Marianne Martus, Mary Morris, Gina Murphy, Jennifer Nolan, Paula Phaneuf, Sue Quackenbush, Mark Stapleton, Bernie Thibodeau, and Amy Thomas.

I also thank the many readers of this manuscript for their encouragement and wise suggestions: Lora Becker-Cook, Barbara Brownyard, Buddy C., Karen Casey, Dawn Champanois, Angie Cosma, William Crowthamel, Pam Gerber, Ann Greaver, Allison Hoff, Harriet Hunter, Ginna Jordan, Janet Kierstead, Jane Molbert, Annabelle Nesbit,

Pam Robbins, Mary Siebert, Coleen Travers, Janice Weber, Marianne Wendt, and Lisa Wilber.

Special thanks to my editors, Teresa Spencer and Anita LeBlanc, who made the book readable and logical, without losing any of the "juice." Kudos to the talented Susi Clark who designed the gorgeous cover and book interior. Also, thank you to Carly Catt for her proofreading genius. Thank you, team, for creating a beautiful and accessible book!

Finally, I'm grateful to my family for permitting me to share our stories: my mother, Cece Wakem Mohlman, an avid reader and connoisseur of language; my father, the earthy, charming, and eccentric Ted Mohlman; and my sisters and brother. I dedicate this book to the memory of Jane Stallings, my spiritual mentor; and Susan Morales, my dedicated and wise therapist.

Preface

May we be at peace. May our hearts remain open.
May we awaken to the light of our own true nature.
May we be healed. May we be a source of healing for all beings.

—Ancient Buddhist Prayer

You probably picked up this book to find a solution to a nagging problem, likely one that's been bugging you for a while. Maybe you're experiencing an ongoing conflict with a loved one or a grudge against a boss. Perhaps you find yourself challenged by your own or another's health problems. Sometimes it's a dream or goal you are drawn to but just can't seem to achieve. Finally, let's not forget the visceral feelings of threat prompted by personal financial woes or world disasters.

Too often your problems appear to only get worse. For example, you get passed over for a job you know you're qualified for. Then you're passed over again. You wouldn't be human if you didn't begin to lose hope and nurse a grudge. Boom! Your heart closes. Reacting to these problems with ongoing bitterness can paralyze you into thinking there are no solutions and all is lost.

But all is *not* lost. What if you could find a way to dissolve your frustration and open your heart to the wisdom of your True Self in every problematic situation? From this place of strength, you can find peace of mind, leading to just the right solution. For example, you might approach your boss with an assertive plan or request. No matter what happens, you accept the results, knowing the best outcomes are on the way. If you continue to reject your fearful thinking and connect with your True Self, something even better often appears, for example, a sudden promotion or a better job.

If you find this hard to believe (and, trust me, I did too at first!), please experiment with the ideas I'm offering and notice how you begin to find a peaceful and courageous approach to your troubling situations.

Your True Self Has Your Back

What is this True Self I'm referring to? It's the divine *you*, deep inside, that guides you through the world with love and wisdom. Although this True Self has never left you, it may have been hidden by heart-closing fears, resentments, and self-criticism. Fortunately, you can remove these barriers by opening your heart to Loving Energy, thus revealing the power of your True Self.

It's not as hard as you might think. In fact, you've already experienced many heart-opening moments of your own. It's just a matter of noticing and cultivating receptivity to them. Here's a story about one such moment in my life.

Many years ago, my third husband and I took a trip out west. Having realized too late that I had married the wrong man, I was miserable the entire time. My stomach hurt constantly, but when I went to the ER, they found nothing wrong. There *was* something wrong, alright, but not with my stomach. I just hadn't been able to face it.

One afternoon late in the trip, we pulled up to a gift shop bordering Jenny Lake in the Grand Tetons. As soon as I entered the shop, I heard a bell-like voice filling the space with song. I just had to know who the singer was! After the shopkeeper told me about Kate Wolf, I immediately bought her tape. From that day on, Kate's music would accompany me as I journeyed out of a hellish life into one of beauty and peace.

With the sweet music still in my head, I exited the shop, made my way to the shore, and found a rock to perch on. Sitting quietly, I watched as the sunlight grazed the water, reflecting back the white-tipped mountain peaks. The image held my gaze. For one long, beautiful moment, I forgot the turmoil of my strangled dreams and baffling, troubled life.

As I stared, the white peaks beckoned to me, seeming to offer another way of thinking, of looking at the world.

New, surprising feelings came to me in a warm, kind voice: *Believe! Trust! Your dreams are still possible. The past is over. Begin anew now.*

Tears welled up in my eyes as I grappled with this unexpected invitation. Taking a leap of faith I didn't know I had, I believed. I trusted. Suddenly, my old feelings of shame, guilt, and hopelessness began to disintegrate.

After that day, I started receiving amazing gifts. First, I found sobriety and a Loving Energy greater than my fears. Then, a therapist helped me overcome the barriers that had been closing my heart: codependency, perfectionism, and people pleasing, to name a few. As I continued to grow, I found *A Course in Miracles (ACIM)*, a spiritual text that teaches how to choose Love over fear in every circumstance.

These resources and many others have given me the certainty, deep down in my gut, that when hardships come my way, I can open my heart to Loving Energy. This Love dissolves the fears blocking access to my True Self. Connected with my center of wisdom, I find peace of mind and the courage to take the proper actions, if any are necessary.

My experience, and that of millions of others, suggests that we can claim our True Self and live the life of our dreams by embracing two vital practices:

Connect your heart with others. It's crucial to find other like-minded people to share your growth and challenges. In such non-romantic relationships, you often find the unconditional Love you've been seeking. Connecting your heart with others involves seeing them as fellow travelers doing their best, just as you are. Imagine approaching every interaction with Love instead of mistrust or criticism. Rather than taking offense when loved ones disappoint us, what if we focus on their true, loving self and cut them some slack? Of course, when necessary, we set firm boundaries, but without bitterness.

Open your heart toward yourself. Can you picture replacing your negative self-talk with positive thoughts? Forgiving yourself for past mistakes? Recognizing when you need a break? It's worth spending some time with this idea, especially if regarding yourself with patience and love instead of self-criticism is new to you.

Will It Work?

As you work at opening your heart, you may doubt that much is changing. The good times sometimes feel rare amidst the challenges. But as you press on, you'll discover little, almost random, miracles of light, of insight, of peace. Such illuminated moments—similar to mine at Jenny Lake—tell you that you're on the right path. For example, you might feel deep appreciation for a former enemy, witness a life-stopping moment of beauty, or act courageously in a situation that used to baffle you. Such glimmers prove that your True Self is there, and it's bigger and wiser than your fears.

We all can grow into the person we hope to be. I know this because I and many others have learned how to dissolve the fears blocking our hearts and live from the power of our True Selves. I offer you the following examples of my life challenges. Although they temporarily stopped me in my tracks, I found ways to open my heart and walk through them with peace of mind and courage.

Relationship failures. After couples therapy, I divorced my third husband, convinced I could never be happily married. A year later, I met Peter, the man of my dreams. Terrified of repeating my pattern of making a man the center of my life, I allowed myself to see him only twice a week. With therapy and supportive, female friends, my heart opened to the possibility of a healthy relationship. Peter and I recently celebrated over thirty years of happy, harmonious marriage.

Worry about loved ones. When my dear friend battled cancer and, later, my fourth husband resumed drinking alcohol, my desire to control others tortured me. No matter what I did, nothing changed, other than my anxiety. Over time I discovered that my sense of security came not from their well-being, but from the Loving Energy of my True Self.

Overwork and perfectionism. As a college professor, I wrestled with fierce professional jealousies, along with a tendency toward overwork and perfectionism. I constantly sought a sense of security through my achievements. Eventually, I learned how to open my heart to others and allow Loving Energy (rather than fear) to lead my efforts. It's one reason I've been able to write this book and *50 Ways to Worry Less Now.*[1] An open, loving heart is a wonderful creative partner!

Dysfunctional family and trauma. I suffered from many of the characteristics found in children of alcoholic parents: heart-closing anxiety, depression, and low self-esteem. I also discovered memories of early abuse, healed its wounds, and forgave those who had harmed me. The healing power of Loving Energy released me from a lifetime of worry about my safety and security.

Poor health and illness. I struggled with back pain for fifteen years. Then both of my shoulders "froze" for two merciless years. With powerful tools to stream Love into my pain (for example, visualization and meditation), I finally recovered. I'm now free of limitations and in excellent health.

Isolation and loneliness. Instead of trying to live as an island of self-sufficiency, I now enjoy the Love and care of women who keep my heart open and full. I know in my gut they will have my back, even if the worst of the worst happens. And I will do the same for them.

Alcohol and drug dependence. For many years, marijuana and alcohol were ruining my relationships and inhibiting my power. I've now been clean and sober for over three decades and have helped (and been helped by) hundreds of women recovering from alcohol and drug addiction.

Although your own challenges may be different from those mentioned here, I know you too can access the loving power and wisdom of your True Self. After practicing this way of living, you'll find that no matter what life throws at you, you can dissolve your fears and frustrations to find a peaceful, courageous way through it.

Concerns about Growing into Your True Self

As you begin your journey, you may have some doubts and resistance to change. That's okay. Once you begin, however, please don't give up. The key is to stick with it, while accepting your reactions with patience and kindness. Here are some common apprehensions you may encounter.

The number one concern about opening our heart to others is that we'll become *weak*—that people will trample all over us. Indeed, the opposite is true. Connecting with the Loving Energy of our True Selves gives us great courage.

For example, after reflecting on and healing our own part in a conflict, we may decide a relationship is no longer good for us. We're able to set and maintain boundaries with such people, but without resentment. Our open heart sees that, just like we sometimes do, they've been acting out of self-centered fear. This is where I affirm, *Open heart, firm actions.*

Another common concern has to do with facing your hidden feelings. What if those ugly, deep-seated fears come bursting forth all at once and you can't handle it? Fortunately, that hasn't been my experience. In fact, my painful feelings have emerged at a manageable pace, and only when I gained the capacity to handle them. Please know that with each new layer of discovery and healing, you'll strengthen your ability to grow through it.

You might also wonder if my referencing Loving Energy is an attempt to make you believe in God. It's fine if you don't, and it's fine if you do. I honor your own conception of a power that helps you overcome fear and limitation. Many of my friends connect with Loving Energy through nature, yoga, meditation, mentors, and many other sources. I've personally learned much from Buddhism, Native American rituals, Christian teachings, and a variety of other wisdom traditions.

Finally, let's talk about commitment. By now you probably realize that growing into your True Self requires sincere dedication. Here's what I see as the essentials for successfully opening your heart to become a loving, wise, and peaceful person.

- *Stay awake!* Refrain from substances and habits that numb your feelings. It's almost impossible to connect with your True Self when you're dulling your emotions and spirit.
- *Hold hands while crossing the street of life.* Choose healthy, open-hearted people as friends and mentors, and gather regularly for fellowship and encouragement.
- *Use specific growth practices.* Flow Loving Energy into your heart and mind to reduce your mind's fear and negativity, and to connect your True Self with that of others.

Yes, it's a lot to commit to and take in. Yes, it requires vulnerability, bravery, and trust; but the process is worth it. Opening your heart to yourself and others will give you access to your True Self and the joy you have been longing for.

My Hope for You

I hope that this book and my other writings provide you with a bank of positive ideas to use when you wish to open your heart, redirect your fearful thoughts, and get to know your true, loving self. You'll never want to live any other way!

Summary

- We're here to move *away from* a life dominated by heart-closing fear, resentment, and criticism, and *toward* a life of open-hearted Love, acceptance, and compassion—for ourselves and others.
- When we open our hearts, we can access the wisdom and courage of our True Selves.
- We open our hearts by allowing Loving Energy to dissolve the fears that block our hearts.
- Opening our hearts to our True Selves brings us peace of mind, courage, and loving connections with others, no matter what challenges we face.
- Overcoming fear-based living requires practice and the support of others.

For Your Consideration

Throughout this book, I'll invite you to pause at the end of each chapter to consider how the ideas apply to you. You may answer all or only a few of the questions. Pick the ones that feel best now. Then either write or draw your responses. Later, you may wish to revisit your reflections to see what has changed or stayed the same.

Before continuing to read, take a moment to identify the challenges you're currently facing.

1. Pick your most troubling situation and list the feelings and concerns you have about it.
2. Now describe how you would like to feel inside about this challenge.
3. Finally, describe how you hope to respond to the situation the next time you encounter it.
4. Reassure yourself that you will find a way to feel and act as you wish. I will be right here with you as we open our hearts to the healing power of Loving Energy.

PLEASE NOTE: This is difficult, brave work, and many overwhelming feelings can surface. If at any time you uncover something too disturbing to face on your own, please consult a mental health professional immediately.

CHAPTER 1

Open-Hearted Living

Life is so generous a giver, but we, judging its gifts by their coverings, cast them away as ugly or heavy or hard. Remove the covering, and you will find beneath it a living splendor, woven of love, and wisdom, and power...Everything we call a trial, a sorrow, or a duty, believe me, that angel's hand is there, the gift is there, and the wonder of an overshadowing presence... Courage, then, to claim it, that is all!

—Fra Angelico

As this quote states so eloquently, there's a gift to be had in every "trial, sorrow, or duty." This was certainly hard for me to believe as I faced my own life challenges. Over time, however, I've made a consistent effort to trust the "angel's hand" and the "wonder of an overshadowing presence." This power helped me dissolve the ugly fears and worries covering the gifts awaiting me: my True Self, a "living splendor, woven of love, and wisdom, and power."

As I've continued to face my life challenges, I've often wondered why they happen. *Why can't everything just be smooth and easy? Is there some punishing force causing all this trouble? What's our purpose here anyway?*

As I pondered these questions, I sought an answer from my friend, Paul, someone I consider a metaphysical sage. For years, he had shared profound truths in our *A Course in Miracles (ACIM)* group, even as he journeyed with grace through life-threatening cancer. So, one day I had a quiet moment with him and asked, "Paul, why do you think we're here? Is it just to find happiness, or is it something more?"

He replied simply, "I've come to believe it's about *opening our hearts to one another*, period." This response resonated so deeply with me that I made it the theme of this book. Here's why.

An open heart connects us to our True Selves: the source of intuitive wisdom, loving compassion for ourselves and others and, most importantly, *joy*. As Shelby John puts it, joy is "the brick and mortar of our lives, a lasting inside job. It's the place we arrive after years of practice, commitment, and sacrifice. True joy is when despite all the craziness happening in life, even with all the heartbreak, grief, disappointment, anger, and sadness, you are solid on the inside."[2] This part of you, the unchanging, beautiful essence of who you are, is another way of describing your Love-powered self.

Being able to access this joy, to live from your True Self—doesn't it sound wonderful? You may question if it's achievable. Well, use your imagination! What might your own solid-on-the-inside life feel and look like? First, think of situations where your heart opens naturally—seeing the smile of a loved one, hearing a favorite melody, experiencing unconditional love, or feeling gratitude for the gifts and kindness you've received. In such golden moments, we behold only the shining, open heart of our True Selves and others. Whatever seems troublesome or wrong in our world just fades away.

Alas, such naturally open-hearted moments can be few and far between. Why don't we live in this joy-filled, peaceful state all the time? It's because years, decades, even lifetimes of glass-half-empty thinking have closed our hearts tightly and painfully. In short, our fears and frustrations have barricaded our hearts, effectively blocking access to our True Selves.

I've come to believe that it's just as my friend Paul suggested: *We're here to learn to open our hearts.* How do we best discover why we've closed them? By using our life problems as opportunities to face our fears, defensiveness, and criticism, and to choose Love, acceptance, and compassion instead.

Fortunately, with guidance and conscious effort, we can wake up to—and change—our fearful patterns and thinking. This next story illustrates how my friend Jada closed her heart as she faced difficulties in caring for her ailing mother. When she realized that her negativity was causing damage to herself and her relationships, Jada made a powerful choice to open her heart. In the process, she healed old fear-driven patterns and gained a renewed confidence in her True Self.

Open-Hearted Living in Action

The difficulty began when Jada's eighty-year-old mother required extensive care during her slow and painful recovery from hip surgery. Even though she had the responsibilities of full-time employment as well as a husband and child, Jada stepped up to become her mother's sole caregiver.

Over time, Jada began to resent her sister for not providing more help with their mother. She added this affront to the litany of past conflicts with her sister, and her heart closed with negativity. What could she do to break out?

The solution to Jada's unhappiness was not found in listing her grievances, or even in getting advice on actions she could take. (You're already thinking of some, right?) No, the answer was for Jada to transform her closed heart to loving openness.

Although Jada's True Self was always there ready to give her insight, she wasn't yet able to connect with it. She just kept on pushing through her fatigue and anger. Finally, she broke down with intense backaches and neck pain, and was forced to stop and reflect. Given this opening, her True Self prompted her to admit that her constant frustration with her mother and sister was hurting her, both emotionally and physically.

Although still reluctant, Jada acknowledged that she needed help and consulted a few wise friends. After empathizing with Jada's situation, they encouraged her to open her heart to herself—to know that her ugly thoughts and feelings were merely human, fear-driven reactions, and that everyone has them from time to time. These open-hearted responses began to shrink Jada's feelings of shame and guilt.

Next, her friends connected Jada with tools known to open the heart. For example, they suggested she visualize a new, desired future where all her troubles were resolved. Concentrating on the glass half-full, Jada imagined having the time and resources to care for both herself and her mother. She saw herself rested, comfortable with her mother's situation, and feeling loving toward her sister. Throughout the long days and before she fell into bed at night, she pictured her new life along with the feelings of freedom and joy she would gain.

Another crucial step was to open her heart toward her sister by affirming the positives in their relationship. For example, instead of criticizing her sister, she recalled the kind things she had done for Jada. By focusing only on her sister's strengths, she was trying to accept her, warts and all.

Finally, Jada took responsibility for her resentment by stepping back and asking herself the hard question: *Why do I think I'm the only one who can carry the burden of my mother's care? I want my sister to help, but I'm unable to ask her.* Part of the answer lay in her role as the oldest child in her dysfunctional home. Sadly, Jada had learned that her needs were less important than those of her siblings. Further, she had found her identity in being a caregiver. These now calcified beliefs had caused her to feel trapped, bitter, and resentful as she cared for her mother.

To overcome these patterns, Jada met with a therapist and made time for spiritual study and reflection. She also practiced switching her self-defeating beliefs to positive ones. Soon Jada began to believe she might be worthy of Love, even when she wasn't taking care of others.

Although it took courage and persistence, Jada's world started to change. For example, a friend invited her to a meditation class where she could gain support from other growth-oriented women. Then, out of the blue, Jada's sister began to visit and help their mother more often.

What had started as a troubling problem resulted in goodness for all involved. Most important, Jada learned to overcome life challenges by opening to the Loving Energy of her True Self and connecting with the wisdom of others. This experience gave her courage and confidence to face and overcome other disturbing situations at work, in her family, and with her own health.

Jada's story illustrates how open-hearted living requires vulnerability and honesty. This may seem like a tough path. But if you're reading this book, you're probably already dealing with some difficulties. Why not try a different way through them?

Choosing an Open Heart

We choose our joys and sorrows long before we experience them.

—Kahlil Gibran

After reading Jada's story, you can see that Loving Energy is a primary force for healing any life challenge. This energy is a highly personal, yet very real force that each of us grasps in our own way. The vitality of our spirits is real. The connection between our spirits is also real. However, we can't see that vitality or touch that ephemeral connection. It's a Love beyond the physical plane.

Given the shortcomings of our three-dimensional world, people try to describe this Love with images they can understand, for example, Loving Power, God, Buddha, Allah, Holy Father, Mother Mary, Gaia, Great Spirit, or Guardian Angel. Others might imagine it as a higher power, Universal Inspiration, Divine Mind, or Oneness. Some find inspiration in nature, movement, writing, or meditation.

Regardless of how we think of this Loving Energy, opening to it is vital to empowering our True Selves. We open our hearts to funnel Loving Energy into our lives, and then send it back out to the world. I believe it's what we're made for; it's our job while we're here.

I created the two images on page 9 to portray how we can either close or open our hearts to Loving Energy. On the left is the person with a closed heart and on the right is the person with an open heart. The images of hearts and stars surrounding the figures represent Loving Energy, always waiting and desiring to be expressed through each person's life. This energy fuels our True Selves!

Notice how the person with a closed heart has puffs of worries and resentments around their head and the jagged edges of dark, negative feelings around their being, blocking the entry of Loving Energy. Finally, notice the brick wall hiding their heart, the essence of their True Self. With so many impediments, it's no wonder only a tiny dribble of Loving Energy can enter their life.

In contrast, the person with an open heart has an unrestricted flow of Loving Energy coming into their life. As it blesses them, they direct it out to serve others. Every time a troubling situation closes their heart with negative thoughts and emotions, this person chooses to access Loving Energy. In turn, the bricks walling off their True

Living with an Open or a Closed Heart

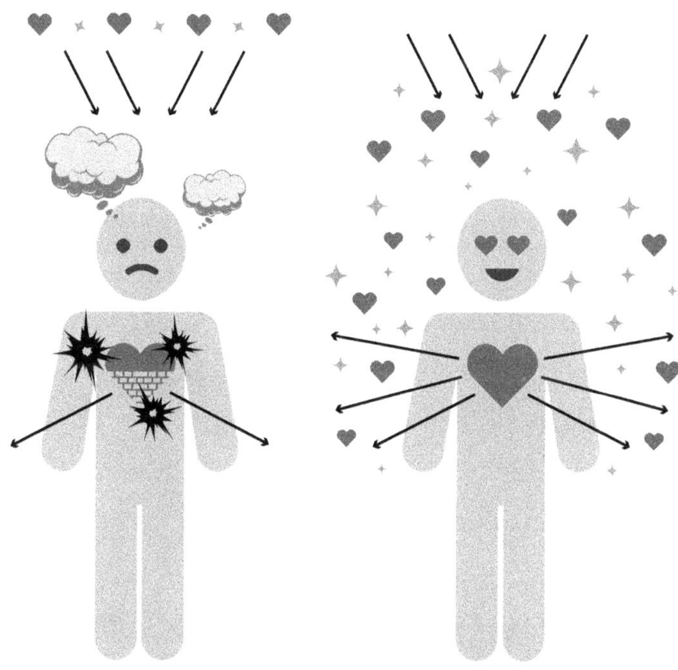

Person with a Closed Heart

Person with an Open Heart

Self dissolve, providing full access to its wisdom, courage, and loving peace.

Thinking back to Jada's example, we see how she began as the person with a closed heart, with cloudy resentments toward her sister blocking her mind from solutions. She also suffered from the jagged edges of fear, guilt, and physical pain.

Fortunately, Jada received a flash of enlightenment from her True Self and sought solutions. Notice that the solutions did not arise through immediate actions to fix the situation itself. No. Her amazing progress came from working on herself—letting go of her fears and resentments so that she could access the Loving Energy of her True Self. In the end, she opened up to compassionate, gentle care for herself and loving feelings for her family.

Who wouldn't want such amazing results in the face of a troubling situation?

Loving Energy Fuels Your True Self

Let me emphasize two important points about your True Self. First, it is your *real nature*, always there, waiting for you to acknowledge it and live from its nurturing care. Second, *nothing can threaten or ruin it*—nothing from your past, present, or future. In other words, you may think you're a failure. You may feel broken and even worthless. The truth is, however, that your True Self—the solid-on-the-inside part of you—remains intact and beautiful, no matter what.

Really. The core of your being—your True Self—is warm, peaceful, loving joy.

We access our True Selves, and all the potential for loving connection it provides, by opening our hearts to Love. Opening our hearts to honest reflection. Opening our hearts to change. Opening our hearts to the struggles of others, and opening our hearts to ourselves.

The results are beautiful, but it's not easy getting there. Opening your heart can bring up painful memories. It may compel you to examine problems you've been pushing aside. Even if this happens, please don't stop trying to discover your True Self.

Closing this book now is a decision to keep your heart closed. It's your choice; maybe you're not ready. But think about it. What will happen if you decide it's too risky or too much work to open your heart? What if you continue to live in worry, regret, and resentment? *Oh, it hasn't been so bad*, you tell yourself. Not bad enough to make such a radical change, anyway.

Again, it's your choice. But remember Jada's physical breakdown? Her destructive thought patterns contributed greatly to her health crisis. Believe me, closing your heart creates life-threatening health conditions, while living with an open heart promotes good health.

An Open Heart Promotes Health and Peace of Mind

If you have aches and pains, aging concerns, or are dealing with an illness, it's well worth your time to learn to live without the stress caused by a fearful, angry, closed heart. Research indicates that negative mental states are just as damaging to heart health as smoking.[3] Further, people who are often angry or hostile are 19 percent more likely to get heart disease.[4]

You may wonder how this is possible, but it's true and it's documented. Most professionals lay the blame on the way our attitudes distort the truth. As author Sonya Collins writes, "Stress is not a reaction to an event but rather to how you interpret the event."[5] She uses the example of the false belief, *If I don't work late every night, I'll get fired.* Along with this belief goes the lie, *I'm stuck and there's nothing I can do.*

Remember how Jada felt trapped by her belief that her mother's care came before her own well-being? Such fear-fueled beliefs increase the adrenaline flow of the fight-flight-or-freeze response. Over time, this causes the body to break down with symptoms such as chronic pain, bowel problems, and heart disease. Jada's moment of awakening was, in fact, due to her extreme physical pain.

Fortunately, the attitudes and fears that negatively impact our health can be turned around by opening our hearts to the Love at our center. For example, the simple act of shifting one's mind toward gratitude has been shown to positively impact health, stress level, and sleep quality.[6]

According to studies from the Mayo Clinic,[7] people who worry less have better physical health, lower risks of stroke or heart disease, and higher overall survival rates. They also have better emotional health, less depression, more harmonious relationships, and are better-equipped to solve life's problems.

The connections our open-hearted selves make with others can vanquish one of the greatest health threats of all—isolation and loneliness. Popular author Brené Brown writes that people who enjoy loving, supportive friendships have greater longevity, better health, more happiness, and stronger resilience in the face of troubles.[8]

Finally, the practice of open-hearted living is especially important for peace of mind today. Our world is on edge. Hiding away in fear might seem to be the answer, but fear closes our hearts to our own potential and that of the world. The act of opening our hearts is one of bravery, and the Love that results is a protective balm for our bodies, minds, spirits, and our planet.

An Open Heart Paves the Way for Loving Connections

You become what you surround yourself with.
Energies are contagious.

—Lisa Becker

We don't live in a vacuum. Most of us interact with others, at least occasionally. If we want to grow into open-hearted, joyous people, there's no way around it: we need other people—particularly those who are farther down the growth path—to show us the way and cheer us on.

This was certainly true for Jada, who began her journey in a state of closed-hearted, resentful self-pity. After finding help from others, Jada was drawn to a mindfulness meditation group where she found new, hopeful friends.

Such connections can be a major source of joy as we stop using criticism and suspicion to distance ourselves from others and allow a little bit of Love into our hearts. Once this flow of Love begins, it keeps on coming—when we keep our commitment to remain open. Soon we're able to reach out to give the same kind of Love to others, as shown in the picture of the person with an open heart. Notice how they have arrows going both inward and outward, indicating that they can not only receive Love but also give it to others.

As crucial as such connections are, you may believe that you can't rely on anyone else. With that mindset, finding loving, healthy people to guide and encourage us can be challenging. In my alcoholic home, I was the youngest, lost in the shuffle as my mother tried to deal with my father's drinking. Growing up with this lack of support, I soon concluded that I was the only one I could depend on.

As an adult, I became fiercely independent, convincing myself that I didn't need anyone's help (except that of my current lover, whom I often made into my higher power). As an island of self-sufficiency, I certainly couldn't acknowledge my pain, except perhaps in a drunken stupor. Denying my emotions was much easier. Finally, after divorce number three, I was compelled to take a long look at my life.

After I quit drinking, I faced the dreaded moment when my psychologist suggested that I join a women's Twelve-Step group. Although it made sense (especially in my case!) to avoid the complications of male attention, I had no idea how to interact with healthy women. Further, I couldn't imagine accepting such support with no strings attached. It was truly a foreign concept. I had allowed plenty of men to "take care" of me, but only when I pulled the strings.

I steeled myself and attended three meetings a week, cold turkey. Fortunately, the women in my group were welcoming and kind. Although I was wary for a long time, I eventually accepted the fact that they had no agenda other than to help me stop drinking, if I wished to do so. Finally, after six months of hearing my recovering friends talk about their loving sponsors, I dared to ask a kind woman named Beth to be my sponsor. I could hardly believe it when she said yes and gave me many hours of her undivided attention to help me work the Steps.

As I began to find my True Self, I learned that my worth had nothing to do with my accomplishments, reputation, marriage, finances, or where I lived. My worth was within me—my solid-on-the-inside True Self. Eventually, I learned to open my heart to this reality by saying this mantra over and over: *only Love establishes my worth*. Knowing that I am grounded in the purity of Love frees me to be an open-hearted person with full access to intuitive wisdom, happy connections, and joy.

You may remember that I listed Guardian Angel as one of the many ways to describe Loving Energy. Perhaps the sober women who taught me about Love were my own guardian angels. Today, I often call such people "Love in skin." Ironically, these angels aren't always who you'd expect, such as family members you think *should* love you. You'll know your own angels because they are the perfect people who appear at just the right time. I'm so happy to be one of the lucky ones, reaching out with Love to each of you!

Serendipity and Angels

When we open our hearts and let go of our fear-driven need to control, our True Selves often attract a bit of magic into our lives. Such miracles that appear out of the blue might be called *serendipity*. Some people refer to them as providence, a "coincidence where Love remains anonymous," or God moments. Regardless of what we name them, we've all had such experiences that defy logic, events perfectly timed to bring us exactly what we need.

Perhaps you've experienced the hand of serendipity as I did many years before I got sober. During my graduate studies at Stanford, I attended a lecture by the highly respected educational researcher, Jane Stallings. As she talked about her studies of effective teaching, I felt a kind of magnetism radiating from her, a combination of charisma and intellect, with a dollop of subtle sensuality. I knew immediately that I wanted to work with this amazing woman. To my surprise, Jane soon hired me to assist with her research on teacher improvement.

During grad school, I spent every evening at a local bar. This seemed like normal behavior to me, but not to Jane. She often phoned at night about some work detail, only to find me less than coherent. One day, Jane gently suggested there was something unsettled in me. Underneath those words I heard, *There's a part of you that's broken, and it shows.*

It shows? I thought I was handling everything, juggling all the plates. But Jane's comment pierced my illusion that attracting men, earning good grades, and being well-liked were hiding my pain.

As I grew under her angelic influence, I was inspired to become an educational researcher, professor, and author. Jane's mentorship changed my life in many ways, but her biggest gift was sending me audiotapes of Gerald Jampolsky's *Love Is Letting Go of Fear,*[9] a simplified explanation of *A Course in Miracles (ACIM).* Listening to those tapes set the stage for my journey to open my heart, recover from alcoholism, and begin transforming my self-defeating patterns.

Since the recovery stage of my life began, I've received other serendipitous gifts. For example, at a meeting I only rarely attended, I met my fourth husband. On another occasion, I heard three people in the same week mention Colin Tipping's *Radical Forgiveness.*[10] I immediately bought the book, and it prompted me to heal my anger toward my father. Finally, I was guided to the perfect editor, typesetter, and proofreader for *50 Ways to Worry Less Now.* These are just a few examples of the beautiful serendipity that an open heart can draw into your life.

Who knows why these magical moments occur? Many call it the work of God. Students of *ACIM* would say they happen when we let go of our fearful thoughts and open our hearts and minds to Love. My friend Kasey Claytor's book, *The Light of Grace*,[11] offers an intriguing portrait of how this mysterious force might work.

Grace, a newly minted angel, is assigned as a life guide to four humans from different historic eras. She takes her role seriously as she watches over them and provides loving help when necessary. For example, she enters their thoughts when they pray, meditate, or savor a scene of beauty. At such moments, they often receive an uncanny insight leading to greater fulfillment and happiness.

But Angel Grace offers other help too. For example, she temporarily comes to earth as a priest named Father Timothy. Garth, one of Grace's charges, is instantly drawn to this priest who helps him find a way through a path that seemed permanently blocked. After Father Timothy disappears, Grace continues to guide Garth as he becomes one of the great spiritual teachers of his time.

Maybe Jane, Beth, and the many others who have helped me heal were guided by some type of angel. Who knows? Whether we call it an angel, Loving Energy, God, higher power, or something else, we know it's a source of unerring guidance and miracles. I think I'll just follow Iris DeMent's advice in her song "Let the Mystery Be."[12]

Although there's an awful lot I've yet to learn, there is one thing I *do* know, deep down to my toes. Loving Energy is available to you and me when we open our hearts to it. My first glimmer of it was at Jenny Lake in that mountain-reflected message of peace and hope. This loving force has remained with me ever since. As you travel the road of open-hearted living, I hope you discover the same plentiful Love in your life.

Summary

- Facing our life challenges can help us find happier ways of living.
- We can resolve many difficulties by rejecting negativity and opening our hearts.
- We access the power of our True Selves by allowing Loving Energy to dissolve the blockages closing our hearts.
- Our True Selves are the center of our wisdom, courage, and Love. It is the essence of who we are and will never leave us.
- Open hearts promote health, vitality, and caring connections with others.
- Serendipity is one of the ways we experience the hand of Loving Energy in our lives.

For Your Consideration

To solidify your insights, I invite you to ponder some (or all) of the following questions. You may wish to periodically revisit your answers. As you continue reading, you may be surprised by the changes in your answers.

1. Which worries, fears, or conflicts may be blocking your heart?

2. Select one of these for this exercise. Put the troubling situation on hold and visualize what your life would feel like if this situation were fixed. Enhance this image with as many loving, positive feelings as possible. Whenever you're tempted to worry about the situation, switch your thinking to this image.

3. Which people have served as angels in your life? How did they help you?

4. Who do you turn to when you need open-hearted comfort?

CHAPTER 2

What Closes Our Hearts to Love and Hope?

I guess you really did it this time...
Did some things you can't speak of.
Oh, who you are is not where you've been
You're still an innocent.

—Taylor Swift, excerpts from "Innocent"

This Taylor Swift song portrays so vividly how my promiscuous past closed my young, tender heart. Yes, I did many things I couldn't speak of, and they tortured me, as at night I lived it all again. Fortunately, my spiritual growth has opened my heart to Love, reassuring me that I am an innocent, and that my True Self shines brightly like a string of lights.

But I didn't learn this lesson until I was an adult. Unfortunately, the people in charge of my early care returned my trust with disappointment and neglect. Although it took many years of therapy and recovery, I am so grateful I no longer believe I'm unworthy of Love.

Perhaps you too grew up feeling full of fear, anxiety, and shame. Many of us did, as our caretakers were often flawed by their own closed-hearted fears. Here we'll explore the experiences and beliefs that have hidden our True Selves (as shown in the image of the closed-hearted person in Chapter 1, page 9). We'll also begin learning how to remove those blockages so we can open our hearts to joy, wisdom, and peace.

Before we start, however, I must warn you that understanding what has closed our hearts is only the first step of many. Beware of falling into the trap of thinking that identifying the causes of your pain will make them go away. Caught up in this "analysis paralysis," you may spend so much time in the past that you fail to do the necessary work to change your self-defeating behavior in the present.

As I navigated my twenties and thirties, I felt like everyone else got the rulebook for finding happiness but me. Satisfying relationships, peace of mind, and confidence—where was my piece of that pie? As I sought Love in all the wrong places—trying to be the person I thought others wanted me to be—I went from one disastrous situation to another, discontented, disconnected, and feeling like a failure.

I thought something was wrong with me, and I hated myself. That's partly why I began numbing myself with drugs and alcohol. I even tried what many call the "geographic cure," moving to places like Brazil, Hawaii, and Germany.

Unfortunately, the physical and emotional fallout from my failed marriages, escalating drug use, and general sense of misery followed me everywhere.

It eventually became obvious that I couldn't address my problems until I stopped using mind-altering substances. When I started recovery and therapy, I was relieved—no, astounded—to discover that I was *not* a defective person, unworthy of loving care. Rather, the adults who were responsible for my well-being had taught me to shut down my heart.

This story from my early childhood is a good example. At age five, I had an appendicitis attack, and no adult was there to help. I rolled around on the floor in desperate pain as my seven-year-old sister watched in horror. I don't know how long the agony lasted, but it felt like hours before my mother finally returned from shopping and rushed me to the hospital.

Subsequent experiences like this convinced me that I could not count on others for anything. Depending on myself to get my needs met seemed like the only way to survive. But this isolation closed my heart even further, especially when my self-centered efforts to find happiness and care failed. For many of us, living with neglect and other negative influences caused us to invent a whole new self: the fake ID.

Closed Hearts Need Protection: The Fake ID

When our hearts are closed to our True Selves, we're left with no choice but to invent a new self, one that can more successfully duck the slings and arrows of daily life. This fake ID is constructed early on for self-protection. Some call it the imposter self or, as I did in my last book, the "invented self."

Sadly, believing that to be loved we must be who others want us to be blocks access to our open-hearted True Selves.

For those of us who grew up in troubled homes, a fake ID was a much-needed survival strategy. To build my sense of security, I watched people who seemed happy and imitated them. For a while, getting good grades and being a good girl did the trick. Then I moved on to boyfriends and early sexual adventures in hopes of finding Love and acceptance.

I constantly sought something outside of me to fill the empty space inside where only fear and self-doubt lived. But none of it really worked. My heart only closed further, leaving me alone and deeply enraged. After my first divorce, I discovered booze and marijuana and used them to erase my pain. Eventually, even that didn't work.

You see, the irony of the fake ID is that it sets us up for failure. It feels like a way to get along in the world while protecting ourselves from hurt. But this strategy backfires because it cuts us off from one of the best parts of ourselves—our emotions.

In my case, I had no idea what I was really feeling. Therefore, I couldn't share my needs with my lovers. Instead, I could only respond from my fears, for example, by accusing them of not understanding me. Without emotional honesty, each relationship ended in frustration and boredom. When this happened, I bolted and went in search of yet another man's affection to fill the emptiness inside.

Another problem with my fake ID was the belief that I was only liked or loved because of the person I pretended to be. This deception spawned constant worry that if anyone knew the real me, they'd leave immediately. In other words, I figured that my real self must be complete garbage.

In a nutshell, presenting a fake self to the world can leave you with anxiety, self-deception, resentment, jealousy, low self-esteem, plus any number of physical ailments. The chaos can seem so confusing that it's almost impossible to hear the voice of your True Self. If you're lucky, you may get the occasional flash of insight that causes you to wonder if there is another way to live.

There *is* another way. Please remember that deep inside, you are an open-hearted being of light and goodness. As you learn to relinquish your fake ID and live from your True Self, your joy will follow.

Countering Our Damaging Whispered Lies

The fake self has set up a long list of mantras to protect the fortress of our closed hearts. I call them *whispered lies* because they are quiet, insidious, and false. When fear's voice dominates our minds with scenarios of impending doom or past shame, it blocks the light of Love trying to enter our lives. Our whispered lies might sound like this:

- *I always fail when I try something new.*
- *I'm sure to be rejected if I reach out.*
- *I always do something to wreck my chance at success, so why try?*
- *If only they would do things my way, we wouldn't have a problem.*

It's okay to admit that we have these thoughts. I do too! In fact, that's why I wrote both *50 Ways to Worry Less Now* and this book: to free us all from the tyranny of such whispered lies so we can live open-hearted, happy lives, fully connected with our True Selves.

Once we acknowledge the existence of our whispered lies, we can learn to change them. For example, I recently became extremely self-critical after making a scheduling mistake. I couldn't believe I had double-booked myself and was quite upset. When I heard that nasty voice asking, *Why are you so stupid?* I realized I had a choice to make: keep listening to its abuse or change it.

One of the best ways to reject our whispered lies is to redirect them to a positive thought. Such thought-switching is simple: when you notice a negative thought, you simply think about anything positive instead. Before starting the exercise, choose the positive thought you will use: an affirmation (such as *All is well* or *My essence is goodness*), a prayer, or a peaceful image of a rose or a nature scene. Then, when you notice that upsetting voice in your head saying, *I can't believe I did it again*, switch over to your positive thought, for example, *All is well.*

Wouldn't it be great if that was all there was to it? Well, I'm sorry to say that one switch is rarely enough to overcome a lifelong habit of negativity. In the case of my recent bout with self-criticism, I needed to redirect my thoughts several times in a single minute. But when I kept at it, I found my heart opening with loving self-acceptance.

Another way to dampen the effect of our whispered lies is to acknowledge how ridiculous they are by laughing at them. My latest episode of self-criticism reminded me of how the "Master-Beaters Club" was born many years ago. While having coffee one day, some friends and I began talking about the internal voices that constantly criticized us, telling us we were bad people, couldn't change, or weren't worthy of loving care. Those whispered lies were eating away at the foundation of our True Selves.

Suddenly, one woman said, "Well, let's just call ourselves the Master-Beaters Club!" We all looked at her and broke into raucous laughter. By giving it such a silly name, we had already weakened fear's voice and opened our hearts to ourselves. Ever since that day, I can quickly reject my self-criticism with a good laugh about our special club. I can then claim, "No more master-beating for me!"

Adverse Childhood Experiences Can Close Hearts

I seek a future different from the past.

—ACIM

Let's admit it. Even in an ideal family, big and little hurts happen. These wounds leave us with a script of heart-closing whispered lies. For example, my friend recently shared how not being invited to the neighborhood birthday party left her with the lie, *I'm not good enough to be included.* In therapy and recovery, she discovered how that belief and others had closed her heart to her beautiful True Self. Now she is one of the most loving people I know!

My own awakening to the damage caused by my childhood experiences came soon after I began therapy. While watching a TV ad showing a smiling, happy family sharing Christmas dinner, I felt my stomach constrict. My breath momentarily stopped. Then it all came to a head, and I blew up, yelling, "That's not how it was at my home!" Since I was alone and there was no one to vent to, I wrote this:

> "I'm the youngest of four sitting at the table at Christmas dinner. My legs dangle. My feet in clean socks and patent leather shoes tap the chair legs. We sit, waiting for Dad to come home. Mom's tense, moving back and forth between the kitchen and dining room, fretting over peas, turkey, and gravy. Our grandmother is quiet, reserved, and disapproving as she observes the scene. Something dark and unspoken thickens the air, but we all pretend it isn't there. Finally, Dad arrives with a slam, boots muddying the carpet, his drunken roars filling the room. I sink lower and lower into my chair, willing myself to be invisible. *This isn't happening*, I tell myself. *I'm not here.*"

So many of us have harsh memories of such ugly scenes, birthed by our parents' fears and unhappiness. Although we knew we were supposed to be happy, we more often felt hurt and confused. Such experiences rocked our foundation and launched us on a search for security, spawning a whole new generation of heart-closing whispered lies:

- *If only they would act better, I could be happy.*
- *I must keep myself safe at all costs.*

- *I am not worthy of Love or care.*
- *If I don't perform well, I will be abandoned.*

Another layer of dysfunction that lies on top of many family problems is how adults handle ongoing issues. Many times, they try to cope by never talking about or even acknowledging the trouble, as was the case in my family. Ignoring the elephant in the room opens the door to whispered lies, as children try to make sense of an unpredictable, scary world. They can't help but think, *Why is everyone sad, but pretending it's all fine? It must be me. I did something wrong. I have to fix it somehow.*

Outside of the home, negative social interactions can also close our hearts. Bullying, social ostracizing, and nasty words from teachers, friends, or boyfriends are only a few of the painful experiences that contribute to persistent and damaging problems in adulthood.

The Adverse Childhood Experiences (ACE) study[13] found that people who grew up with damaging conditions—inside and outside the home—are at significantly greater risk for depression, panic, anxiety, promiscuity, alcohol/drug abuse, smoking, and/or eating disorders. On a hopeful note, the ACE study found treatments such as journaling, mindfulness meditation, therapy, self-care, and neurofeedback to be effective in easing the negative beliefs formed in our childhoods. Simply put, these approaches help dissolve the whispered lies closing our hearts, opening up access to our True Selves.

In my case, I was raised in an alcoholic home with drunken shouting matches, emotional neglect, and sexual abuse. No wonder I became alcoholic, promiscuous, anxious, and depressed! When I finally learned about the connection between my problems and the adverse experiences of my growing-up years, I must admit I felt hopeless, convinced that I was irreparably broken. The harmful patterns had begun so long ago. How could anything ever change?

However, there *was* hope. Many of my new friends had been attending Adult Children of Alcoholics and Dysfunctional Families (ACA) meetings and shared how helpful they were. So, I decided to attend ACA, too. At my first meeting, I felt a giddy sense of relief as I saw others willing to face and banish their old elephants in the room. If they could use the Twelve Steps to overcome their fears and insecurities, so could I.

It was at those meetings that I heard—and believed—these empowering words: *I'm not to blame for my childhood, but I* am *responsible for healing its effects.* Embracing this truth helped me see that I was not doomed to repeat the patterns launched in my youth. If I took the risk of opening my heart, perhaps I'd find a treasure there.

Being a Highly Sensitive Person Can Close Our Hearts

About fifteen years ago I discovered the empowering fact that I am a highly sensitive person. And I'm not alone. Eileen Aron's[14] twenty-five years of research indicate that about 20 percent of the population shares this trait. It might sound like a negative aspect of one's personality, but it has an upside. You'll be happy to hear that sensitive people are quite respected in many societies, where they often become community advisers and sages.

Unfortunately, those around me didn't see it as a strength. For years, I was told I was thin-skinned or too high-maintenance. I honestly didn't understand what they meant, but I knew I reacted differently in many situations. I took offhand comments and jokes personally. Loud noises and bright lights bothered me. I found socializing and pretending to be funny exhausting. By contrast, my closest ally in the family—my fearless, outgoing sister—seemed to have no cares at all. I eventually assumed that something was just plain wrong with me.

Feeling isolated by my differences, my critical inner voice often berated me with whispered lies. To make things worse, my boyfriends and former husbands also accused me of being too sensitive and insecure.[15] Of course, my fears chimed in that they were right, reinforcing my need to close my heart and live from my fake ID.

Dr. Aron writes that highly sensitive people…

- are quite sensitive to external stimuli (loud noises or bright lights),
- become drained of energy after intense socializing,
- worry excessively and are easily overwhelmed,
- reflect on things more than others, and
- feel things intensely.

In our extroverted Western culture, being highly sensitive isn't always understood or valued. That's why some of us feel as if we're on the outside looking in, watching those who seem to move through life easily, and whispering to ourselves, *What's wrong with me?* To hide our awkwardness, many of us resort to the fake ID—shutting down our pain, pretending to be okay, and closing our hearts to our dear True Selves.

The healthiest path for us sensitive types is to discover and nurture our true goodness; for example, by switching our thoughts from *There's something's wrong with me* to *I'm okay just as I am, sensitivity and all!* Then we're in a position to take good care of our tender selves.

If you think you might be a highly sensitive person or have a loved one who is, take the quiz on Dr. Aron's website and check out her blog, *Comfort Zone.*[16] If you do relate, here are a few suggestions for self-care:

- Remind yourself that your sensitivity makes you creative, empathetic, and loving.

- Reduce your exposure to loud or dramatic input delivered by news programs, social media, or argumentative friends/family.
- Schedule downtime to rest, meditate, read, and renew after lots of work or social activity.
- If bright lights and loud background noise bother you, avoid them.
- Sleep enough, eat well, and limit caffeine intake.
- Treat yourself to the enjoyment of beauty as you take a walk or savor a sunset.
- Hang out with loving people who like you exactly the way you are.

Insight into the effects of living in a dysfunctional family and my naturally sensitive nature enabled me to see my divorces and addictions not as evidence of irredeemable flaws, but as simply misguided attempts to find Love and security. I was able to let go of self-condemnation and cherish the innocence of my True Self. Most importantly, I began to heal my old self-defeating patterns.

Negative Patterns Can Close Our Hearts

Every journey into the past is complicated
by false memories of real events.
—Adrienne Rich

If you're on a growth path, chances are you've discovered some patterns that are bumping up against your dreams of satisfying relationships, success, or health. For example, you might find it hard to speak up for yourself at work or with your life partner. Perhaps you're prone to outbursts of anger that scare your loved ones.

When such problems crop up, it's helpful to know you are *not* fatally flawed. Rather, it's likely that some old self-protective habits are keeping your heart closed.

In many families of origin, day-to-day life was all about staying safe and reducing the family chaos. Some children became high achievers. Others took care of everyone else. Still others got lost in the shuffle, hiding in the corners. Some deflected the tension and conflict with humor or distraction. Each of these tactics relied on the illusion of control reflected in the whispered lie, *If I do this, they won't be so upset, and I will be safe and loved.*

Even as we approached adulthood, many of these habits worked pretty well in school and work, where it seemed easy to mold ourselves to the situation at hand. However, the patterns we thought were protecting us eventually turned out to be damaging and even deadly, especially to our relationships.

Navigating adult relationships requires honesty and vulnerability—in short, an open heart. When we continue our heart-closing ways, we find ourselves repeatedly facing problems that seem to get worse no matter what we do—divorces, lost jobs, illness, or addiction, to name a few. Waking up to the futility of our efforts, we may get a nudge from our True Selves telling us it's time to give up our old self-protective habits.

Because we've been blindly obeying our heart-closing patterns, it's essential to begin to identify them. In *Stage II Recovery*,[17] Earnie Larsen outlines six common ways that we sabotage our happiness. You may immediately identify with some of them and think, *Oh, that's me! I'll never be able to change.* First of all, ease up on the critical self-talk. Secondly, don't worry. If you're awake, open-hearted, and connected with healthy advisers and friends, you can unlearn the habits that have blocked Love for yourself and others.

Here are Larsen's six negative patterns with examples of associated whispered lies.

> *The Caretaker.* Caretakers feel responsible for the happiness of others; they try to rescue people, often to the detriment of their own self-care. *I can't be happy if everyone else isn't okay. I can't let anyone down; I must make things better.*

The Martyr. Martyrs believe life is a struggle and they're the victim of an unfair world. They don't believe they deserve fun or pleasure. *Life will never work out for me. I always lose out, no matter what I do. I can't handle life.*

The Perfectionist. Perfectionists can't stand making mistakes, have a low tolerance for unpredictability, and are often critical of others' incompetence. *Everything has to be perfect for me to be okay. If I work hard enough, I can fix this. I hate failure.*

The People Pleaser. People Pleasers constantly seek approval. They need to keep everyone happy; therefore, they put their own needs last. They have trouble saying no, can't handle conflict, and often feel hurt. They lack confidence in their own opinions. *For me to be safe, everyone must like me. I can't object to my loved one's nasty words. I can't say what I think because people will hate me.*

The Workaholic. Workaholics put the completion of tasks ahead of their relationships and health. They feel guilty when not working and feel they never accomplish enough. *I must get it all done, or my life will fall apart. I can't take time for myself or others because there's just too much to do. I am nothing without my work.*

> *The Tap Dancer.* Tap Dancers constantly test the limits, avoid commitment, and often skirt around the truth. They always have an escape plan in case things don't work out to their liking. *No one can pin me down; escape is my only security. I bet I can get away with this, just to show I can. I won't commit to therapy or recovery.*

When I first read this list, I identified as a Perfectionist, Workaholic, People Pleaser, and Tap Dancer. As a Perfectionist, I completed an advanced degree at Stanford, but my whispered lies had me in knots of stress, leading to drug abuse and promiscuity.

As a Workaholic, I ignored my family and partner by spending all my time studying or working, which contributed to the failed romantic relationships. As a People Pleaser, I had no idea how to identify or state my needs. I was terrified of conflict and just went along, pretending that everything was fine. No wonder I left each of my three marriages in a state of confused frustration!

Finally, my Tap Dancer pattern had me traveling all over the world, leaving a relationship whenever I got bored, and frequently changing jobs and degree programs. I think the first time I didn't try to skate past a commitment was with my sobriety.

If you can identify with any of these patterns, it's important to recognize that each one has its strengths as well as its problems. For example, once you let go of needing to please everyone, you still have the gracious social skills you've cultivated as a People Pleaser. When you manage your Tap-Dancing tendencies from a place of courage rather than fear, you can still take advantage of your resourcefulness and spontaneity. When your workaholism relaxes, you'll find you can still get a lot done. It's just a matter of removing the cutting, harmful side of the pattern.

Please remember that you *can* change the habits that have been closing your heart and sabotaging your relationships, health, and happiness. I see people do it every day. An easy first step is to start switching your internal dialogue from criticism to kindness.

Self-Compassion Soothes the Wounded Heart

At this point in the chapter, you may be feeling a bit shaken up—that's a good thing. Perhaps you're feeling thrown off your game because you're starting to loosen the foundations of your old, familiar habits. Or, you might be considering new ways of living.

Coming face to face with our need to change is not fun. It's difficult to admit that we have contributed to our present difficulties by allowing old habits to close our hearts. But have no fear! You can comfort yourself right now with self-compassion.

According to researcher Kristin Neff, "Having compassion for yourself means that you honor and accept your humanness...You will encounter frustrations, losses will occur, you will make mistakes...and fall short of your ideals...The more you open your heart to this reality instead of constantly fighting against it, the more you will be able to feel compassion for yourself and all your fellow humans in the experience of life."[18]

Instead of just ignoring your pain with a stiff upper lip, Neff suggests you tell yourself, *This is difficult right now. How can I comfort and care for myself in this moment?*

Self-compassion is the exact opposite of self-criticism. Nor is it self-pity, thinking, *Poor me! I'll always be this way.* Finally, it isn't excuse-making, believing, *I have this pattern because of [fill in the blank], and it will never change.* Self-compassion means you open your heart to yourself by offering kindness and understanding when confronted with personal failings. Remember, you're human.

So, how do we give ourselves self-compassion? Neff suggests we talk to ourselves as we would a hurting little sister or brother: *I'm so sorry that happened to you. It would hurt me, too. Just know that I love you and I am always here.* Such loving words give great comfort.

Since I'm often driven to take on big projects and then get stuck, I get many opportunities to practice self-compassion. For example, when I can't figure out something on the computer, my Perfectionist voice immediately whispers, *What the hell is wrong with you? Other people can do this so easily!* Since I know this voice so well, I've learned to stop and soothe myself by answering: *Yup, it is frustrating to get stuck. I hate it. Remember how we've been here so many times, and eventually, we figured it out? Let's take a couple deep breaths and try one more time. If it doesn't work, we can take a break and come back to it later, or ask for help.*

Whenever a situation scares me or shakes my security, I notice my closed heart and move into self-compassion. Sometimes all I need is to take a break by going for a walk, meditating, or resting. When I return to my task, my True Self is once again available to help me find a solution.

We Are *Not* Our Old Patterns

Our closed hearts lead us to do and say things we deeply regret. Even after we've attempted to make amends, we may feel that there's no more goodness left in us. Not so! Regardless of the mistakes we've made, our solid-on-the-inside part is still there. We can claim this truth at any time by reasserting that we are perfect, innocent beings who cannot ruin our True Selves.

At one of my early Twelve-Step meetings, I heard someone say, "God don't make no junk!" Even though I squirmed at the word "God," I desperately needed to believe something good about myself. Remember, I had disconnected from my True Self and thought I was nothing without my fake ID—my invented, people-pleasing self. Further, shame over my past sexual and drug adventures had closed my heart, leading me to believe that I truly *was* a piece of junk.

To my relief, I discovered that my recovery buddies had felt similar pain and shame. But what shocked me most was that they no longer felt that way. In fact, they happily proclaimed freedom from their old selves and embraced their true ID by affirming, "God don't make no junk!"

Recognizing this truth releases us from fear's darkness and brings us into the sunshine of our True Selves—a wonderful place to live! It's just as Taylor Swift's song suggests, "I'm an innocent." And you are, too.

To close this section, I must share this darling quote I recently found on Facebook: "A new approach to self-care: Talk to myself the same way I talk to my dog (or cat). 'Hey, sweet girl. Look at that beautiful belly! You're so clever!'" Great advice!

Keep reading to learn how to discover the golden light in your center by freeing yourself from limitations, fear, and self-defeating patterns.

Summary

- Many of us invent a fake self to give us a feeling of belonging and security. Over time, all this pretending restricts our ability to love, sabotaging our relationships and lives.
- Whispered lies are internalized critical messages aimed at ourselves or others. They always limit our willingness to give and receive Love.
- Adverse childhood experiences can create many self-defeating and painful conditions, but these can be reversed with heart-opening therapies and practices.
- Although being a highly sensitive person is ultimately a gift, we struggle against it in our early years, feeling different from others. Over time, we learn to take care of ourselves and cultivate our gifts.
- Our past experiences have taught us coping patterns based on fear and a need for security. Unfortunately, these negative habits block access to our True Selves.
- Through self-compassion and consistent honest effort, we can leave behind our destructive patterns and find Love for others and ourselves.

For Your Consideration

If you wish, take a few moments to reflect on how the ideas presented here apply to you. If you've found areas you'd like to change, reassure yourself that you can do it—with effort and support.

1. What are some of your frequent whispered lies? How do you overcome them?
2. In what ways have you created a fake ID, and how have you begun to discover your True Self?
3. Which early experiences might have contributed to your life difficulties?
4. Are you (or is a family member) a highly sensitive person? What do you see as the pros and cons of being highly sensitive?
5. Which survival strategies or patterns helped you feel secure in your youth, but have caused difficulties for you in later years?

CHAPTER 3

Opening to the Wisdom and Power of Your True Self

If you had not fallen, then I would not have found you,
Angel flying too close to the ground.
Love is the greatest healer to be found.
—Willie Nelson, "Angel Flying Too Close to the Ground"

The image of the angel crashing to the ground is all too familiar for those of us who have faced loss, failure, addiction, codependency, or other hardships. There we lay, broken-winged, our closed hearts too heavy to rise again, too grieved to take another risk.

However, if we're open and willing to try, the curative power of Loving Energy soon appears—perhaps in the form of a helpful friend or inspiring teacher—and we rise and rise until we fly on toward our dreams. Then we reach down and help the next angel repair their broken wings, so they can soar in loving freedom with us.

In this chapter, we're learning to connect with our True Selves—a place of calm, internal wisdom, unfettered by whispered lies or external circumstances. This center of Love is courageous, generous, and powerful enough to fulfill your dreams. Plus, your True Self has wings!

Transforming the patterns blocking your heart takes commitment and consistent practice, but it is totally worth it to feel calm, secure, and content in your life. In my experience, such growth is a fine dance, balancing honesty versus denial, and isolation versus connection. Every day we choose between the despondency of our old patterns and our new open-hearted life.

Four Strategies to Open Your Heart

In *50 Ways to Worry Less Now,* I offer four life strategies to dissolve the fears and patterns blocking access to our True Selves. Any time I run up against a life challenge (chronic pain, illness, worry about a loved one, conflict with friends or family, or unsettling working conditions), I use these four strategies to remove the fears closing my heart. They've never failed to connect me with the peace, wisdom, and joy of my True Self. I hope they will do the same for you.

Let's use Jada's situation from Chapter 1 to illustrate the process. Recall that Jada felt trapped by her need to take care of her mother after her hip surgery while also working full-time and caring for her family. She was frustrated and angry that her sister had not pitched in to help her. The last straw came when Jada was laid up with neck and back pain that prevented her from taking care of anyone but herself.

Get Honest. In the quiet of Jada's inactivity, a split second of honesty allowed her to admit her feelings of being trapped and to wonder if there was a better way of dealing with her situation. Such moments of clarity often come from our True Selves (unless we're dulling its influence with mind-altering substances or habits).

Claim Power. Jada's willingness to reconsider her old ways opened the door to a Loving Energy greater than her limiting patterns. This possibility first appeared in the form of a few wise friends she could confide in. Soon, Jada began to consider the idea that her True Self could lead her to the right solutions if she continued growing.

Make Choices. First, Jada began to envision her relations with her mother and sister as completely healed, with her own health restored. Next, Jada committed to use growth tools to transform the patterns limiting her peace and happiness.

Use Growth Practices. In this step, Jada opened her heart to her sister by focusing only on her strengths. Next, she questioned why she felt she could be the only caregiver for her mother and family. To dissolve the whispered lies closing her heart, she used therapy, meditation, and other tools. As a result, Jada found new ways to care for herself, her sister, and her mother.

Now let's delve into each of the four life strategies in greater depth.

Strategy 1. Get Honest

At this point in this book, you probably realize that you've been unable to fix your most troubling situations all on your own, and that perhaps there is a power—a source of wisdom—greater than your own thinking. That's what happened to me when I first honestly admitted I had a problem with alcohol and marijuana.

Strategy 2. Claim Power

Although I've been writing here about the power of Loving Energy, it took me quite a while to warm up to this idea. At my early recovery meetings, I knew I had wrecked my life by continuing my drinking and promiscuity into my third marriage. But my closed heart couldn't fathom that any kind of power, higher or not, could help straighten out my life. Plus, I bristled against the God terminology tossed around so casually at meetings.

Before getting sober, I had made two attempts at becoming a Christian, both of which failed. First, I simply could not admit that I was basically sinful, as they insisted. Second, I did *not* trust the male God figure that was supposed to take care of me. Why wouldn't this one hurt me, as my father and other males had done?

However, there were few other options for getting sober in 1986, so despite the God language, I kept going back to meetings. Eventually, I found a measure of peace in the suggestion that I didn't have to accept anyone else's concept of a God—I could develop my own. So, I stuck around, grateful for the care I experienced and intrigued by the atmosphere of hope.

As I observed the obvious joy and sense of freedom in the people at meetings, I couldn't help but wonder if what they called a "higher power" was, in fact, responsible. If so, perhaps something greater than myself *could* lift me out of my misery. And maybe I didn't need to nail it down quite yet.

I kept at it by continuing to attend meetings and therapy. Then came the day when I held my six-month medallion and figured *something* had to be keeping me sober. Although I couldn't imagine such power coming from a traditional God figure, I felt an undeniable Loving Energy coming through the care and wisdom of my sober sisters.

This initial glimmer of Love helped open my heart and drew me to explore spirituality further. Soon, some friends invited me to a Unity congregation in Warren, Michigan, led by Jack Boland, who was in Twelve-Step recovery. He was the first preacher whose words from the pulpit didn't set off my bullshit detectors. Instead of talking about sin or punishment, he spoke only of Love, and, to my surprise, he often referred to the teachings of *A Course in Miracles (ACIM)*, the centerpiece of the spiritual life of my grad-school mentor, Jane.

ACIM, along with many other wisdom traditions, teaches that each of us is an individualized expression of Loving Energy, sinless and pure, and that our loving open hearts are joined with all others, now and forever. Sound familiar?

Further, our lives mirror what's inside us. Thus, what I see in my mind reflects outward to create—yes, *create*—my experiences. You might wonder, *How in the world does my mind create my experiences?* Well, it's a matter of choice and persistent use of growth practices—strategies three and four!

Strategy 3. Make Choices

We can choose our future. Sounds outlandish, right? But it works, especially when our wishes involve the nonphysical world, such as mending relationships or being of service to others. In such areas, Loving Energy can be marshaled to produce the most amazing outcomes—as long as we don't get too prescriptive. In other words, when choosing our desired future, it's good to leave some wiggle room for a bit of serendipity and miracles.

You've probably heard of the Law of Attraction, which says that when you align your thinking and actions with your dreams, you can attract them into your life. Simply stated, what we hold in our minds produces in kind, a key idea in recent research on positive thinking and manifestation.[19]

I first experienced the power of intentionally choosing my future when I joined a Master Mind group, one popular application of the Law of Attraction. In Jack Boland's protocol,[20] we affirmed our trust in Loving Energy to help us change, and then each of us made a request for our desired future. We confirmed each person's request before going on to the next member. At the beginning of each day during the following week, we visualized each person's desire as coming true. Of course, one of my requests was to be in a healthy and happy relationship. However, I didn't specify with whom or when or how. I just trusted the process.

After several weekly sessions, the miraculous demonstrations began. I could hardly believe what I was witnessing! For one, I met a man who was healthy and fun, and instead of instantly merging my life with his, I lived alone for the first time. We took our relationship slowly, and today Peter and I have been married for over thirty years. That's some power, eh? More miracles: I landed the job of my dreams, stayed sober, and gained a healthy group of female buddies. Other group members experienced similar joys, such as finding new jobs and healing damaged relationships.

Although everything about my life was improving, I still needed to consistently use growth practices to overcome the negative thinking that often closed my heart.

Strategy 4. Use Growth Practices

Whatever you hold in your mind on a consistent basis is exactly what you will experience in your life.

—Tony Robbins

Let's face it. Part of being human is to fall into negativity, anger, and self-criticism, among many other unloving states. Even after all these years, I am not free of such fear-driven misery. When this happens, however, I have a big toolbox of practices that flow Loving Energy into my heart and mind. You've already read about some of them here: thought-switching, meditation, prayer, and connecting with other loving people.

Such tools fill our minds with positive thoughts, leaving little room for the negative to enter. Free of our fears and old patterns, our hearts open and our lives begin to improve. But how do we keep up these positive habits and continue to thrive?

Let's begin by looking at general self-care as a tool for growth. We all know that babies get cranky when they've not had enough food or sleep. It's the same with us. When I'm hungry, angry, lonely, or tired, my thinking gets out of whack. In Twelve-Step recovery, these four states spell HALT, a reminder to stop and take care of ourselves. When I notice my nasty attitude (swearing at other drivers is always a tip-off!), I ask myself if I'm feeling hungry, angry, lonely, or tired. Then I take care of those needs and move on.

In a similar vein, we can think of growth practices as spiritual and emotional self-care. When we've consistently filled our minds and hearts with Love, we're more resilient, better able to handle disappointments and tragedies. Plus, when others need our loving care, we can provide it while still maintaining our own healthy boundaries.

Here's another reason we need to consistently use a variety of growth practices: our old patterns can be difficult to dislodge. We are, after all, reprogramming a lifetime of mental and emotional habits. For example, if I have a falling out with a friend, I'll probably need several tools applied over a few days to let go of blaming them and look at my part. With help and consistent efforts to replace fear with Love, I'll eventually find a way to mend the relationship, or perhaps let it go.

When we continue our commitment to growth, we can reframe even our biggest life challenges as opportunities to face and release negative patterns. I'm proof. Along with the successes in my first years of my sobriety, I faced several daunting challenges. I badly sprained my ankle, had major surgery, and injured my back. After a year of couples therapy, I divorced my third husband.

Such challenges could have easily tipped me back into hopelessness. But that didn't happen because I had continued to use many growth practices. In addition to regular attendance at my Twelve-Step meetings and therapy, I also meditated, prayed, and said affirmations. As I used these tools consistently, I opened my heart further to the light of my True Self.

In my third year of sobriety, I joined my sponsor, Beth, in her *ACIM* study group, and encountered this image of Love as a light: "The light is in [you] now…It is the only thing you bring with you from your…Source. The light cannot be lost…The light within you is sufficient."[21]

Given this new awareness, I began to see the light of Love not only in myself but in others. To this day, when I see a woman walk into a Twelve-Step meeting, no matter her ragged state, I instantly perceive the shining light of her True Self. Looking back at my first years of recovery, I now realize that those early angels, my sisters, saw this same light of Love in me when I couldn't yet see it in myself.

Speaking of the light of Love, here's an example of how a friend used the affirmation, *Be the light,* to reduce her concerns about conflicts in her workplace.

> "I love how in your talk you referred to spirituality as 'a light. A light inside us. A light for others to see.' Here's how I've been using this idea in my daily life. I was so excited to be able to pass a drug test, and get a real job, benefits, good pay. But then the place turned out to be very toxic. Gossip, fighting, and plenty of non-recovering alcoholics. I became sucked in very quickly.
>
> I was fairly new to recovery and hadn't learned many tools. I would sit out in my car every morning and pray to go in there and be the light. To shine bright and help the hurting souls in there. I prayed for God's will and the strength to not get sucked into the drama.
>
> Afterward, I would go to meetings and share my pep talk about 'being the light.' How it was helping me at work, reminding me to be the change. To spread compassion and love to those who are still sick. How I had to remind myself over and over. For example, I would be in the middle of the bickering, and I'd whisper under my breath, 'Be the light. Be the light.' Then I'd put up my boundaries and walk away.

> Next thing you know, other people in the program were talking about it. How they would find themselves in situations and would pray for the light. The light to rise above. For the light inside themselves to shine bright. What a gift to help others by sharing how I shine the light of spirituality. And, by helping others, we help ourselves."[22]

This story illustrates how opening our hearts to Loving Energy can heal any situation. What impact might we have if we try to be the light in the lives of each person we encounter? For example, when visiting a sick friend, we can focus on the light in them rather than the illness; when hearing gossip, we remain silent and shine light on the person being criticized; when discussing the news, we quietly shine Love into the world rather than focusing on the darkness. In such ways, we can increase the flow of Love for all.

Connecting with Your True Self

Try seeing yourself through the eyes of someone who admires you. They aren't connected to your negative beliefs about yourself. All they see is your true glory and potential.

—Jen Sincero

Living in the light of our True Selves isn't complicated. In fact, it's deceptively simple: reduce the fears that close our hearts and turn on the light of Love within our hearts. However, according to most wisdom traditions, there's one thorn, one stickler, that continually gets in the way. Too readily, we close our hearts toward ourselves and the whole of humankind by *focusing on faults and deficiencies* rather than goodness.

Fortunately, there *is* a solution. Because you have complete control over your thoughts, you can change them at any time. First, you need to honestly admit that you're contributing to your negative mood. For example, you might notice you're imagining a painful future or pondering regrets from the past. Sometimes you'll observe yourself being short-tempered; for example, swearing when you drop something. These are clues that our minds have gone on a glass-half-empty journey, spinning tales of woe and resentment—and even more damaging, closing our hearts to life.

When we notice such tensions, we can claim the power to redirect our thoughts from negativity to Love. For example, when my mind whispers to me that I'm not safe, or I'm not getting what I want, I simply ask Loving Energy to help me see things with an open heart. When I notice my mind returning to my fears, I ask again, *Help me to see this with an open heart.* Sometimes the change takes place quickly, sometimes slowly, but if I keep asking, my outlook will change for the better.

Finally, you can practice connecting with your True Self by simply lying on your bed and surrounding yourself with nurturing Love and protection. Sometimes it helps to use a guided meditation on self-love or repeat statements such as:

- *I am a uniquely created and purely innocent being.*
- *My essence—my True Self—is a spirit of Love and care.*
- *My worth is established by Love.*
- *Whatever may have happened in my life, it does not override the truth of who I am.*

Cultivating the ability to see things differently when we are confronted by challenges takes practice and commitment. You might groan at hearing this and wonder if it will really do any good. But it's not just another self-help suggestion to put on the list. Changing our mindset from negative to positive, from fear to Love, from worry to hope, is essential. It's basic. In my experience, it's the only path to peace and happiness.

Okay. I'm in, you say. *So, what's the payoff?* There are many. How about never feeling hostage to your life challenges? How about visualizing loving relationships and receiving them? How about seeing yourself as contributing your best assets to benefit others?

We all have such hopes and dreams, right? They're worth pursuing. The next sections describe more ways to access the power and wisdom of your True Self.

Meditation: Discovering Your True Self

There is nothing more important to true growth than realizing that you are not the voice of the mind—you are the one who hears it.

—Michael Singer

Meditation is one of the fastest ways to connect with the Loving Energy of your True Self. As Ram Dass says, "The quieter you become, the more you can hear."[23] When I mention meditation, however, many reject it, thinking, *I've tried that, but I couldn't empty my mind. It just kept wandering.* In my experience, the goal of meditation is not to completely empty our minds; rather, it's learning how to *notice our thoughts and redirect them* as we choose.

When I first tried to meditate, my guide suggested I sit quietly and observe my thinking. After a short time, he asked me, "Who is now observing your thinking?" It shocked me to realize that if I could sit and watch my thoughts, then *I must be more than my thinking*—an idea I'd never considered. I had always believed I was at the mercy of my thoughts and had no control over my spiraling negativity and fear. Now I was learning to see through my fearful thoughts to find the heartbeat of my True Self underneath them.

The only requirement for meditation is to focus your attention on one thing (your breathing, a mantra, an image), observe how your thoughts stray, and then gently bring them back to that one thing. When the noise of your constant thoughts settles down to that one focus, you begin to connect with your True Self, infinite and always fused with wisdom, Love, and peace.

Research on meditation shows it has a calming effect on the brain, reducing hyperactivity in the areas associated with fear, threat, and trauma.[24] This valuable tool has taught me to direct my mind away from worrying about my problems, and to focus instead on Love—where the best solutions lie.

Even though I know the benefits of meditation, it's difficult for me to do it first thing in the morning. Right out of bed, I dearly enjoy my cup of coffee with my husband, chatting and watching our cat's antics. After that, about half the time I'm off and running. There goes my plan to meditate, right out the door with me!

Given this tendency, I need "training wheels," so I love it when Deepak Chopra and friends offer their twenty-one-day meditation series.[25] It's free, and each one centers on a different theme. For example, a recent series focused on attracting our desires into our lives. In one episode, Deepak was his usual clear self as he explained the Law of Attraction:

> "What we pay attention to will grow. The power source for manifesting our dreams, desires, and intentions is attention. When attention is focused from the level of true self, our desires easily reach fulfillment. Desires that arise from a worried, confused, or agitated mind struggle to be fulfilled. When we meditate, the intentions arise naturally from the silence, and the energy of attraction automatically obeys what the mind desires."[26]

There's another great reason to meditate. Tapping into my quiet, open-hearted self always yields insights, valuable nudges for action, and creative ideas for anything I attempt. In fact, I've found I can't write any of my books or articles without meditating first.

If you too need some training wheels for meditation, download the app, Insight Timer, or check out some of Kelly Hine's fabulous guided meditations. Finally, here's a comical view of meditation from my dear friend, therapist Susan Morales: "How Not to Meditate."

> "Wear your tightest jeans; not the stretchy kind; the ones that pinch at the waist so your midriff folds over and it's hard to breathe. Recall a recent conversation where you felt misunderstood and

> analyze what you should have said. Visualize what you'll do the next chance you get. Find something on your body or clothing to help you fidget, like cleaning your fingernails, picking the pile off your sweater, or winding your hair around your finger. Don't set an intention or an alarm, look at the clock every time you think of it. Focus outside yourself, inhale short and shallow. Tell yourself you can't meditate."[27]

I hope you got a big laugh out of Susan's humor. I sure did! If you struggle with setting aside a big chunk of time to meditate, try short bursts of mindfulness instead.

Mindfulness: The Now Moment

Mindfulness is defined as a therapeutic technique where "a mental state is achieved by focusing one's awareness on the present moment, while calmly acknowledging and accepting one's feelings, thoughts, and bodily sensations."[28] That's exactly what we've been talking about, right? Our best connection with our True Self is right here, right now, in this present moment.

But let's face it: most of us tend to live in the wreckage of our future by fearing all sorts of catastrophes—a sick or injured loved one, disability, poverty, loneliness—the list goes on and on. We worry and obsess as if we could control the future by thinking about it. Ha! Not likely. And guess what? It's no use fretting about the past, either. It's over, *completely* over, and there's no changing it.

This quote from Melody Beattie expresses the idea of mindfulness so well: "One thing at a time. That's all we have to do. Not two things at once, but one thing done in peace. One task at a time. One feeling at a time. One day at a time. One problem at a time. One step at a time. One pleasure at a time. Relax. Let go of urgency. Begin calmly now. Take one thing at a time. See how everything works out?"[29]

Because mindfulness isn't easy for me (maybe it isn't for anyone, at least at first!), I enrolled in Mindfulness-Based Stress Reduction (MBSR)[30] to retrain my wandering mind. This eight-week course, developed at the University of Massachusetts Medical Center and offered all over the world, teaches people to fully appreciate the present by focusing on the body's sensations and movements. One exercise involves taking several minutes to chew a single raisin while savoring the full experience—the texture, taste, and sound. Give it a try sometime. You'll be amazed.

To develop your ability to be mindful, try focusing one hundred percent on what's happening right now, right in front of you. What details do you see? What do you smell? What noises do you hear? What tastes fill your mouth? What is touching your body? How does it feel?

When you're this attentive to the present, you can feel yourself unhinge from distressing thoughts about your past and future. You get out of your head and are better able to enjoy the present. After all, this moment, right now, is the only one we have, right?

By the way, the developers of MBSR have conducted extensive studies showing that mindfulness meditation improves physical health and sleep quality. It also reduces stress, depression, anxiety, emotional exhaustion, and burnout.[31] That's a pretty big bang for the buck!

To sum up: since we can't control the future or change the past, why not just admit it, relax, do the best we can, and leave the results up to Love? Staying in the present moment is a pretty cool way to live—when we can remember to do it.

The Price of Urgency

My mind often whispers, *I've gotta go faster. It will be horrible if I can't get this done on time!* Such urgent thoughts initially scare the wits out of me. Then I recall my propensity for Perfectionism and Workaholism and remind myself, *I'm more than these thoughts, and I can access Loving Energy to change them.*

To recalibrate my exaggerated, negative self-talk, I breathe, meditate, pray, and use mindfulness to connect with my True Self. And then, voila! Those things that just *had* to be done are accomplished effortlessly or at just the perfect time. For example, a changed deadline, or a canceled appointment gives me time for an important conversation.

We pay a big price for our urgency. As some say, we're either "now here" or "nowhere." Our obsession with time blocks our openness to the loving connections and beauty available to us every minute of our lives. For example, while preoccupied with a task carrying a self-imposed deadline, we may only half-listen as a loved one shares their feelings. How sad to miss such an important opportunity to strengthen that relationship!

Another cost of mindless urgency is missing the poetry of an especially beautiful moment, such as a glowing sunset or a gorgeous piece of music. In one of my favorite novels, *The Elegance of the Hedgehog*, Muriel Barbery perfectly captures this kind of bliss: "I have finally concluded maybe that's what life is about: there's a lot of despair, but also, the odd moment of beauty, where time is no longer the same. It's as if...something [is] suspended, an elsewhere that had come to us, an always within never."[32]

An "always within never"—what a fitting image for those golden moments of beauty. Aren't we each a bit of a poet when we let go of our urgency and wake up to what's happening right now, with all its drama and magnificence? In this present space lies the truth of you, your wise and wonderful True Self, available to generously give and receive Love.

The Soothing Power of Your True Self

Those of us with troubled childhoods sometimes find a disturbing event will throw us back into feeling unsafe and without protection. In such cases, we can communicate lovingly with our inner child, the part of us that holds the memories of neglect and abuse as if they were still happening today.

Even as an adult, when things scare me, I sometimes return to the panic and visceral fear I felt as a little girl in an alcoholic home. I'm sure many of you can relate. This terrified part of us needs reassurance, and it's available in the form of the adult part of our psyche—our healthy True Self who can provide loving understanding to our inner child. Many times, that's all it takes—a word of compassion and a visualized hug. At other times, such as when we've been deeply hurt by others, we go to bat for our inner child by setting strong boundaries.

My sponsor, Beth, sometimes tells me to "stay in my adult" rather than reverting to my insecure child state. This advice was especially helpful when we moved my mother into a nursing home. In her partial dementia, she angrily erupted into screams I hadn't heard since I was a child. I froze with terror and barely made it to the bathroom to call Beth. She listened with care and then suggested that I touch a solid object to remind myself that I was here right now as an adult, not a helpless child. As I grasped my wedding ring, I told my inner child that I was right there with her and would not let anyone hurt her. With this technique and Beth's comforting words, I was able to return to my mother's distress with calm strength.

An important part of self-care is acknowledging that we still have some old tender spots—what some refer to as being "triggered." No matter how much healing work we've done, experiencing a certain sharp phrase or attitude from another person can cause us to quickly regress to a child's helpless feelings, sometimes creating an angry eruption. That's understandable, as long as we don't stay there. If we harm others while in this state, we admit we were wrong and make amends.

We're less likely to be triggered if we've been working to keep our hearts open to our True Selves. That means we work daily to keep growing away from fear and toward Love.

Daily Routines to Open Your Heart

Switch your mentality from* I'm broken and helpless *to* I'm growing and healing *and watch how your life changes for the better.

—Reyna Biddy

Sometimes our negativity has us by the throat, whispering lie after cruel lie in our minds. It feels almost hard-wired into our brains. But remember: our negativity is *not* permanent. In fact, experts in neuroscience[33] reassure us that we can substantially transform our thinking from negative to positive. But it takes consistent practice.

That's why we need to establish a daily routine to fill our hearts with Loving Energy. *Why daily?* you might ask. Because our brains are not like computers where we change the program one time and it is done. Over our lifetimes, our minds have learned only too well to be mistrustful, judging, self-critical, resentful, defensive, and afraid. So, it's going to take time and consistent effort to rewire that mess. Here are some ways to build and maintain your open-hearted life.

> *Support.* Try to find people who can serve as mentors for your new ways of thinking, perhaps through Twelve-Step programs (they have them for almost everything), church events, social media support groups, spiritual advisers, or online coaches. To counter my natural tendency to isolate, I meet with my recovery partners at *ACIM* and Twelve-Step meetings at least three times a week. I schedule these meetings in my calendar and give them the same importance as any other commitment. Remember, we can't do it alone!

> *Morning routine.* Start your day with an inspirational reading that connects you to Loving Energy.

Then perhaps settle in for a short meditation (alone or guided) and conclude with a prayer (perhaps the Serenity Prayer) and/or an intention (for example, *Today, my True Self leads me to my best life*).

During the day. Fill your mind and heart with inspiring ideas and people. I listen to uplifting podcasts about people's victories over hardship. I also read daily affirming emails from TUT.com because they're fun, personalized to my dreams, and so positive! As I encounter people, I try to see only the light of their True Selves and treat them with kindness. Finally, I protect myself from emotionally inflammatory people, TV, and other media.

At the end of the day. Before going to sleep, make a gratitude list by listing at least five things, people, or events that you're grateful for. Many people try not to repeat any item from the prior days, which teaches your mind to search out the good stuff for your nightly ritual. In Chapters 4 and 5, we'll learn how to examine and heal the situations that are still disturbing you.

If all this seems like a lot of effort, remember that these routines protect you from falling victim to your whispered lies, anxiety, and stress. Such small investments in your happiness bring amazing results: serenity, abundance, and courage to face your most disturbing situations.

Try a few of these ideas. For example, to cultivate an appreciation for your life, try simply thinking about what you *do have* rather than what you *don't have*. With consistent practice with these tools, you'll be amazed by your open-hearted freedom and your emerging belief that everything will be alright.

The Peace of Perfect Order

How much simpler our lives can be if we only have the faith to accept what happens as a guidepost along a path that is naturally correct.

—Hazelden

I've often written about how our lives are in *perfect order*, that as we work toward open-hearted living, we can rest assured we're always on the right path. This idea can be tough to accept when so many things appear to be a mess. But despite these appearances, I still trust my wise, True Self to lead me along a "naturally correct" path of growth.

I believe this because, when I look back, I see how working through my scariest times resulted in the most amazing outcomes. For example, facing my alcohol and drug use brought me a spiritual path, healthy friends, and a happy marriage. Many years of dealing with back and shoulder pain taught me to accept the things I cannot change and to receive comfort from others. Finally, when I was able to overcome my doubts, I published my first book.

When your mind is consumed with fear about a current life situation, please remember that, even though it doesn't look like it, everything is in perfect order. The loving hand of your True Self is ready and able to lead you out of your difficulty. Later, when you look back, you'll be able to see how those challenges were guideposts for valuable learning along your path. In short, everything is alright.

A few years ago, while watching the TV presentation of *Jesus Christ Superstar Live*, I found a new appreciation for the song "Everything's Alright" as it echoes this same truth: Our lives are in perfect order, guided by Love. So, we can just relax. Here are a few of my favorite lyrics.

> *Try not to get worried,*
> *Try not to turn on to problems that upset you, oh,*
> *Don't you know, everything's alright, yes, everything's fine.*
>
> —Andrew Lloyd Webber and Tim Rice, "Everything's Alright"[34]

Here's what these words mean to me:

Don't dwell on the hopelessness of your problems. Instead, redirect your mind to open-hearted hope, care, and positive thoughts. Focus on what is saving you (your True Self's wisdom), not on what is scaring you (the problem).

You don't have to fix all the problems of the world. Just detach from trying to control other people and things and allow the world to spin on its own. If and when help is necessary, you'll intuitively know how to provide it.

Allow Love to calm your worries. Just close your eyes and relax. Instead of planning and plotting, think of nothing but Love. From this cool, sweet place come insights, inspiration, and solutions for all your problems.

Just imagine relief flowing through you as your True Self's wisdom takes charge of every problem in your life. Even when your troubles seem overwhelming, you'll find the comfort you need. If action is required, your True Self will guide you to it. After things settle down, you can look back and see how your healing path unfolded in perfect order.

Relax. Everything's alright. It really is.

Summary

- We can open our hearts by getting honest, claiming power, making choices, and using growth practices.
- Consistently using growth practices keeps our hearts open and self-limiting fear at bay.
- We can connect with the Loving Energy of our True Selves by switching our thoughts from fear

to Love, asking to see things differently, meditating, and being mindful of the present moment.
- Urgency is an enemy of mindful connection with life and Love in the present moment.
- When triggered, the "adult" voice of our True Selves can calm our insecurity and fears.
- To maintain our connection with the Loving Energy of our True Selves, we use daily routines to flow Loving Power into our minds and hearts.

For Your Consideration

To consolidate your learning, take a moment to ponder the following questions. Respond in writing or as you wish, perhaps through creating images.

1. Which practices have you used to open your heart to Loving Energy?
2. How well have they worked and why do you think so?
3. Which new practices discussed here appeal to you?
4. How might these new ideas be helpful for a current challenge you're facing?
5. What daily routines will you use to build a positive, loving life?

CHAPTER 4

Creating Open-Hearted Relationships

I can leave myself to rot in the past, spend my time hating people for what happened...or I can forgive and forget... It is so much less exhausting. You only have to forgive once. To resent, you have to do it all day, every day. You have to keep remembering all the bad things.

—M.L. Stedman

It takes only an instant to close our hearts to someone. We think our relationship is going along fine, and then the other person says or does something that hurts us. The minute this happens, our fears seize on it, whispering lies such as, *It's not fair! They should have...They should not have...*or *What's wrong with them?* Suddenly, they are the enemy, and we begin to nurse a grudge.

I believe the cause of most unhappiness is resentment, thinly disguised as criticism, disapproval, blame, complaining, jealousy, or envy. Some say holding onto a resentment is like drinking poison and expecting the other person to die.

And, as Stedman's words above indicate, anger tends to eat away at us because we keep reliving and re-feeling the pain of our disappointments and complaints.

Many of us are unwilling to honestly face our unpleasant feelings and instead resort to pretending that nothing's wrong. But unresolved anger doesn't really disappear. In fact, it's inside us just waiting to come out. For example, some people, especially the Martyr types, make snide comments or use sarcasm toward the offending person. We call this "anger coming out sideways." People Pleasers, however, tend to hold in their resentments, fearing a confrontation and loss of approval. As the poison builds up, it simmers painfully inside, just waiting to erupt in a sudden, nasty scene, prompted by the most minor of incidents.

The price we pay for harboring resentments goes deeper than damaged relationships; it is life-threatening. I've already mentioned that people who are often angry or hostile are 19 percent more likely to get heart disease. Further, cardiac patients who remain angry and hostile have a much shorter life-span.[35]

If we want to have open-hearted relations with others and good health, we must find a way to overcome our fears and resentments. First, we stop avoiding the feelings and honestly acknowledge them; second, we connect with the power of our True Self's Loving Energy; third, we choose to become who we want to be in our relationships. Finally, we use a variety of growth practices to accomplish this goal and open our hearts to those we meet along the road of life.

Professional Jealousy Closed My Heart

Many years ago, when I was a professor of education, I formed a grudge against a colleague who I'll call Dr. Smith. She was very popular with her students, and since we shared an office space, hearing her students fawn over her with admiration made me wildly jealous. *She's not so great,* I thought. *I could list a dozen things I do better! I used to get similar feedback from my students. Oh no, I must be slipping!*

When I finally realized that this constant negativity was draining my energy and causing my jaw to clench, I told my sponsor about the situation, hoping to gain a new perspective. After listening patiently, she suggested that perhaps I had been relying on my teaching awards and positive student ratings to give me a sense of security. Well, that was a dose of reality!

Although I didn't like hearing that, I honestly reflected on it and began to see how my Perfectionism and People Pleasing were telling me, *Everyone must love you for you to feel safe and worthwhile. You're the only one who can be on top.* I had bought into the whispered lie that there was a limited amount of appreciation to go around, and if Dr. Smith got more attention, then I could only get less of it.

As I accepted this uncomfortable truth, I realized I needed to do the work to dissolve my whispered lies and open my heart toward Dr. Smith. I began by affirming that each of us enjoys unlimited Loving Energy and security by repeating over and over, *Our worth is established by Love.* Next, I practiced seeing only her goodness, her True Self, rather than the nasty images my fearful mind had conjured. At first, this thought-switching didn't take, and my mind quickly reverted to its private pain and envy. So I tried again, kindly noting my negative thoughts and choosing to see her essential light instead.

After a few weeks of using these growth practices, I began to feel a genuine, open-hearted connection with Dr. Smith, a connection that lasted. When I overheard her students praising her, I felt truly happy about it. The miracle of replacing fear (separation) with Love (connection) had occurred.

And guess what? Replacing such resentments with Love is a twofer! As I open my heart to another, that openness returns to benefit me. In this case, I felt my Perfectionism soften, freeing me from self-condemnation and fear. It was, and remains, a win-win.

Connecting Our True Selves in Relationships

The major block to compassion is the judgment in our minds. Judgment is the primary tool of separation.

—Diane Berke

When we close our hearts to anyone, we separate from them. We focus only on what we perceive to be their flaws and misdeeds, not their True Self. But when we let go of our judgments and open our hearts, we connect with others at the deepest level of loving acceptance.

I created the image on page 82 to illustrate the difference between open-hearted connection and closed-hearted separation. The left side illustrates how our True Selves connect as one, all worthy of Love. In this state, we have easy and constant access to the Loving Energy that dissolves the barriers to Love.

Now take a look at the right side of the figure, where a closed heart separates us from others. In this lonely condition, we see no one as worthy of Love, including ourselves. Even worse, we think we're each on our own, competing for a limited amount of Love that is never enough.

But first, please note the most important word of all—*choice*—in the center of the image. Every time you think of another person, you're choosing to either connect with them or separate from them. Whether you realize it or not,

Choosing Open-Hearted Connection over Closed-Hearted Separation

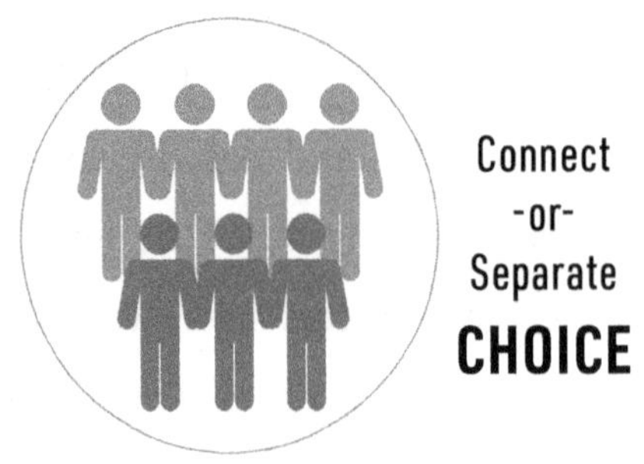

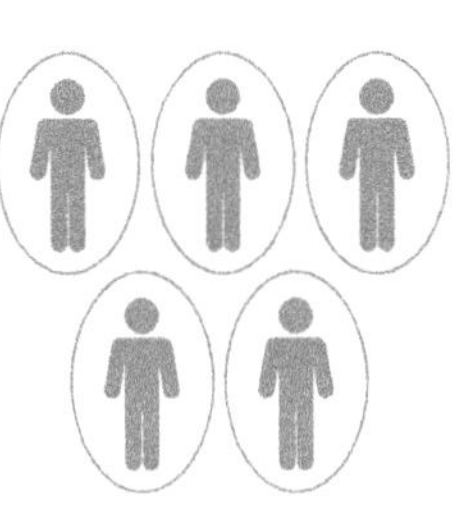

Open-Hearted Connection
All Worthy of Love

Closed-Hearted Separation
No One Worthy of Love

you are deciding if they are worthy of your Love. If they are not, you have closed your heart to them.

On the left side of the image, we are all connected as one on the spiritual level. The way we behave toward others reverberates throughout this universe. If we choose separation, we expand fear and suffering. Offering Love, on the other hand, becomes a healing balm for all.

Barriers that Cut Others Out of Our Hearts

Unforgiveness means holding onto something we reinforce in our minds and make real because we do not want to look at ourselves and how it is that we have contributed to what we see as someone else's problem.

—Jon Mundy

As Rumi wrote, "The fault is in the one who blames. Spirit sees nothing to criticize."[36] As seen in the quote above, our emotional pain is caused in our minds, not by others' actions. It's an inconvenient fact—but it *is* a fact—that what's important is *not what happened*; it's what we're *thinking and believing* about what's happened. Therefore, when we're hurt or disappointed, it's our responsibility to honestly reflect on how we might be contributing to our negative feelings.

Often, our initial reactions in adult relationships are reproductions of negative patterns learned long ago in our dysfunctional families or with others. In Chapter 2, we examined six of them: Caretaker, Martyr, Perfectionist, People Pleaser, Workaholic, and Tap Dancer.

To change these self-defeating patterns, we need to ask ourselves how four main barriers to Love have kept these patterns in place: *How have my Resentments, Self-Centered Motives, Self-Deception, and Self-Condemnation closed my heart to loving thoughts and actions?*[37]

As an example, let's look at how Workaholism can disrupt a family's loving connection. Imagine that one partner complains that the other partner works too much, and that when they're finally home, they're too exhausted and short-tempered to pay attention to the children. Upon hearing these complaints, the working partner's Self-Centered Motives whisper, *If I work* less, *I'll lose the respect of my colleagues, and I couldn't stand that!* Then, Self-Deception chimes in, *I must work this much to keep my job and support my family.*

If this partner doesn't honestly consider the family feedback and face these barriers to Love, they'll end up missing a chance to change. However, by accessing Loving Energy to dissolve the fears blocking their True Self, they can let go of their Workaholism and find a healthy balance at work. With an open heart, they can connect more fully with their family members.

Such changes begin with identifying our faulty thinking and beliefs. Here I illustrate how each of the four fears blocks Love with heart-closing whispered lies and relationship-killing consequences. On the right, we see how Love's truths and benefits emerge as each barrier is dissolved.

Resentment Blocks Love	**Resentments Are Dissolved**
• **Whispered Lies:** *Nothing works out for me. I never get what I deserve. Screw life! I hate them! They shouldn't have done that!* • **Consequences:** Self-pity, distrust, envy, criticism, intolerance, gossip, blaming others	• **Love's Truths:** *I have everything I need right now. Everything is in perfect order; I just can't see it. This person is just as troubled as I am. I can let go of my anger, and take firm action.* • **Benefits:** Acceptance, compassion, generosity, forgiveness, gratitude, setting boundaries
Self-Centered Motives Block Love	**Self-Centered Motives Are Dissolved**
• **Whispered Lies:** *If they get all the attention, then there's not enough for me. I must get this now so I can be happy. I'm more worthy than they are. Other people's needs don't matter.* • **Consequences:** Competitiveness, jealousy, anxiety, impatience, pride, greed, withholding love, inflexibility	• **Love's Truths:** *I am an equal among equals. We're all loved and loveable. I can give care to others, and all of us benefit. There's enough Loving Energy to go around.* • **Benefits:** Satisfying and rewarding relationships, generosity, consideration for and acceptance of others
Self-Deception Blocks Love	**Self-Deception Is Dissolved**
• **Whispered Lies:** *Nothing is wrong. My blow-up wasn't that bad; why don't they understand? If I can change them, then I will be happy. If I try hard enough, I can keep my loved ones safe.* • **Consequences:** Denying problems, anxiety, disconnecting from feelings, justifying negative behavior, trying to control others, health issues	• **Love's Truths:** *I can face myself and others with honesty and care. I can't change people, places, or things, but I can change how I think and act. Loving Energy ensures our security.* • **Benefits:** Honest self-reflection, wisdom, courage, truthful communication, acceptance, emotional security, resiliency
Self-Condemnation Blocks Love	**Self-Condemnation Is Healed**
• **Whispered Lies:** *I don't deserve Love. I'm worthless. I can't handle life. I give up. I'm all alone.* • **Consequences:** Depression, anxiety, loneliness, failure, self-harm	• **Love's Truths:** *My worth is established by Love. My True Self can handle anything. I can join with others to give and receive help.* • **Benefits:** Joy, success, peace of mind, loving friendships, self-compassion

May Transforms Her Relationship with Her Ex-Husband

This story concerns my friend, May, a lovely woman in her forties with two children she's raising with limited assistance from their father. She has a huge heart, beautiful smile, and has overcome too many obstacles to name. With four years of sobriety under her belt, she has created a new, healthy life for her family. However, her alcoholic ex-husband and his family have been a constant irritant.

Since the divorce, they've treated her like dirt. He entered her home without permission, his parents ignored their grandchildren, and he made insulting comments in every phone conversation. Unfortunately, May condemned herself as a horrible person, just as they had told her.

May's story highlights how, at first blush, the problem seemed to be the way her ex-husband treated her. But it was really about freeing herself from long-standing negative patterns that kept her from claiming her power. Fortunately, with a loving sponsor, therapist, and healthy friends, she has learned how to do so.

May began working with me on her old pattern of People Pleasing and its whispered lie, *Since I don't want to risk angering him, I must put up with his poor treatment.* I encouraged May to consider her part in the problem by asking herself, *How was I Resentful, Self-Centered,*

Self-Deceptive, and/or Self-Condemning? Here are May's answers to these questions.

1. **Resentment.** How was I resentful? *I stewed with anger, but turned it on myself, contributing to my physical pain and addictions.*

2. **Self-Centered Motives.** How was I self-centered? What did I do to get my way? *I tried to manipulate him into respecting me by doing things for him. Plus, when I was drinking, I only thought about myself.*

3. **Self-Deception.** How did I deceive myself? What truth did I not want to face? *I held on to the fantasy that perhaps my behavior would cause him to change, but it never happened.*

4. **Self-Condemnation.** How had I condemned and criticized myself? *I believed he treated me poorly because I wasn't worthy of Love. I thought I was a screwed-up person who couldn't get myself out of this horrible situation.*

After sharing with me her insights, May sought therapy to address her complicated feelings and learn new ways of communication. She was lucky to find a skilled therapist who was trained in Eye Movement Desensitization and Reprocessing (EMDR)[38] who helped her work through her negative beliefs about herself and the traumatic aspects of her past. She also stepped up her spiritual practice with prayer and meditation, tried to focus on the positive qualities of her ex-husband and his family, and also claimed the power to stand firm in setting and maintaining reasonable boundaries for their behavior.

After a couple of months, she wrote this note to me: "Now I see my ex-husband may never treat me the way I want. I don't deserve his abusive, nasty words and actions. It's okay for me to set boundaries and enforce them. I have plenty of people who love me just as I am, so I don't need his approval. For now, he can't love us with an open heart."

As of this writing, May continues to remove her barriers to Love through therapy, prayer, meditation, and studying *ACIM*. She recently told me, "I'm becoming an honest girl who says it like it is, rather than a good girl who puts up with poor treatment." This insight has given her the courage to maintain powerful boundaries with her ex-husband and his parents.

Recently I heard her say this profound truth: "I can only claim my True Self's power when I give up the belief that my own fears will protect me." May's courageous growth shows that, with guidance, we can heal the patterns and barriers to Love that no longer serve us. In fact, growing out of our fears is the only way to open our hearts to ourselves and others.

Letting Go of Resentments: Forgiveness

You are already joined in truth to all the people in your life at the deepest level. Even those you do battle with are one with you, beneath and beyond the earthly connection.

—ACIM

How do we make real, lasting changes in our most troubling relationships? How do we conquer our stubborn resentments? It's easier, and it feels justified, to flat out condemn other people's frailties and misdeeds. After all, they've hurt us.

However, if we approach the problem with an open heart, ready to love and be loved, we can admit how difficult it is to be consistently loving. For all of us. Everyone struggles and everyone deserves compassion, even those we "do battle with."

Realizing this truth, we now come to the idea of *forgiveness:* joining our hearts rather than separating. Admittedly, forgiveness can be a challenging concept. Many of us have a negative, knee-jerk reaction toward this word because of our experience with religious teachings. Some of us learned that forgiveness is merely lip service: pardoning someone who has hurt us but still harboring resentment and viewing them as an enemy.

Remember the diagrams of Open-Hearted Connection and Closed-Hearted Separation on page 82? The act of forgiveness is a key component in choosing to connect our hearts in loving unity. In this view, we focus on the open-hearted, loving essence of each human being, regardless of how they've done wrong (or "missed the mark," as in the Hebrew definition of *sin*).

Please know that forgiveness is rarely an instant fix. As many of the world's wisdom traditions teach, it's a *process* of letting go of our barriers to Love and replacing them with loving, positive regard for those who have hurt us. This is a big ask, right?

My friend, Paula, sure thought so! When she read this section on forgiveness, she immediately called me to ask how she could open her heart to her stepdaughter, Lisa. Despite Paula's kindness and her husband's occasional reprimands, Lisa had been verbally abusing Paula for over twenty years.

The situation blew up when Paula refused (for the first time) Lisa's request for a big favor. In her reply, Paula said that, given how Lisa had been treating her, Paula would not grant the favor. The "elephant in the room" they'd all been tiptoeing around was finally out in the open and the finger-pointing began. After a long discussion, Paula and her husband agreed that Paula would leave their home while Lisa stayed for the holiday.

As Paula shared her frustration with me, she wondered how she could possibly forgive Lisa for all the years of abuse, including this latest conflict. I congratulated her on her honesty and courage, empathized with her feelings, and encouraged her to have self-compassion. We both saw a silver lining to her anger because it had prompted her to do something different.

But the question remained: *What should she do now?* Here's where our challenges get tough because, typically, we *cannot* change the other people in a troubling situation. Realizing that, however, is the beginning of healing.

First, we refrain from acting while we soften our hearts to ourselves and all involved. Fortunately, Paula has a strong spiritual foundation, and accepted that only a power greater than her distress could guide her through this dilemma. She began bringing Loving Energy into the picture, affirming that a solution would arise as she connected with her True Self.

She then reflected privately on her part in contributing to the situation: What patterns and barriers to Love had caused her to close her heart? Next, she used growth practices to stream Love into her heart and mind, thus dissolving her old Caretaking and People-Pleasing patterns. This opened the door to new ways of responding.

When she returned home, Paula and her husband had a long, honest talk. They ultimately agreed to invite Lisa to be with them for the next holiday. Although they would do their best to keep their hearts open, they would set and maintain firm boundaries as necessary. I wish them well.

Here's a final image of forgiveness that may help you grasp the idea. Imagine it as giving Love and care to another *before* they've done anything to deserve it. I often think of the word forgive as "fore-give," or "before-giving." Fore-giving is simply looking beyond negative appearances and seeing only the light of another's True Self, no matter what they've done.

Please know that forgiveness does *not* mean we put up with abuse. As I said earlier, we strive for an open heart backed up by firm actions. Still, when we choose to "fore-give," we expand the force of Loving Energy in the world, thus helping to dissolve fear and selfishness.

A Terrifying Conflict

As the saying goes, fear's favorite food is conflict. I believe it. It's tough to mend a relationship without resorting to old methods of pretending there's nothing wrong (stuffing our feelings) or blowing up (to vent those pent-up feelings). It requires honest self-appraisal, powerful wisdom from our True Selves, choosing to respond with Love, and using tools to open our hearts to the person on the other end of our dilemma.

Although personal conflict is inevitable, it still terrifies me. Last winter, I had a quarrel with my niece's next-door neighbor (and sometimes boyfriend), Joe. My not-so-hidden negative attitude toward him had been brewing for some time, as my niece had complained about how he treated her. Since I had been rehearsing his faults, that's all I could see when he offered to help me with my car's dead battery.

After Joe used a jumper cable to start my car, he suggested I buy a new battery before I drive the 200 miles home. I thanked him for his help and said I needed to call home before getting a new battery. He replied, "Why do you need to do that?" I repeated that I needed to call my husband because he does all the car maintenance. Then Joe leaned into me and asked the same question, but more aggressively. When I again said I wanted to call home, he got into my face even more, saying, "You don't really need to do that, do you?" That's when I blew up and said, "Go f—k yourself!"

After my outburst, my heart was pounding, and I felt dizzy. I went into my niece's house, rushed to the bathroom, and closed the door. I reassured my inner child that yes, that had been scary, and our reaction was understandable. But now she had me to take care of her. Then I said a quick prayer and used a 5-4-3-2-1 technique to dissolve the adrenaline flooding my system. Here's how this technique, originally designed to quell a panic attack, works:

First, take a few slow, belly-inflating breaths. With compassion, admit that you're feeling threatened, and your reaction is normal. Then start the countdown.

- Name 5 things you can see around you *(I see a rug, a painting, a window, a door, a wall).*
- Name 4 things you can feel *(I feel my feet on the floor, cool air on my skin, my heart beating, my hands resting in my lap).*
- Name 3 things you can hear right now *(I hear a fan running, people's voices outside, the clock ticking).*
- Name 2 things you can smell right now *(I smell perfumed soap and dinner cooking).*
- Name 1 good thing about yourself *(I know how to help myself through this).*

If you simply can't focus, or if you haven't settled down, take a few more belly-inflating breaths and tell yourself that you *can* calm down. Then repeat the entire process.

This exercise helped me anchor into the present moment where I could connect with my True Self. After settling down, I sought out Joe to apologize, but he was having none of it. And it was too soon; we both were still hurting. All I could do was be civil when I ran into him later that day.

Since that episode, my niece moved in with Joe, and they invited my sister and me for dinner. Thank God, I had several weeks to prepare for the visit. As I reflected on my part in the conflict, I realized that my childhood trauma was part of the problem. My old fears caused me to revert to a helpless child and lash out in anger.

But, even with that insight, I continued to replay and resent his intimidating behavior. I was also afraid that any conversation with him would turn ugly. Feeling stuck, I began talking about these concerns with my sponsor. We determined that if I was constantly imagining another attack, that's probably what would happen.

Then I remembered that I could turn away from my fear-filled projections and, instead, choose to see the best in this man. I spent the next weeks visualizing Joe's pure, true self instead of his past behavior. In essence, I was trying to forgive him. But he wasn't the only one who needed forgiveness. I did too.

At that time, I happened to hear the gifted ACIM teacher Carol Howe explain how we condemn ourselves harshly when we "misbehave." Suddenly, I realized how ashamed I was about blowing up at Joe. I had closed my heart to myself with Self-Condemnation, a very painful state. Given this insight, I began to work with Colin Tipping's Radical Self-Forgiveness—a process for transforming conflicts into opportunities for growth. This tool helped me heal an old resentment toward men who overpower women. With continued prayer, I began to feel sincere love for myself and Joe, warts and all.

As I traveled to my niece's house on the evening of the dinner, I kept my heart open and refused to anticipate an attack. I did, however, reassure myself that if I felt uncomfortable, I could leave the room and take a moment to calm myself. And, if I felt really threatened, I could even leave early.

To my relief, the entire visit was very harmonious, except for one moment when I observed Joe say a few harsh words to my niece. She looked at him directly, clarified what he was asking, and calmly replied. To my amazement, I was able to watch the interaction with no judgment or resentment. Further, I witnessed my niece's ability to take good care of herself. Wonderful!

It's true that dealing with our part in relationship conflicts is not easy. But the alternative is living in a closed-hearted, isolated bubble of fears and resentments. Choosing to separate from the joy of loving connection is a pretty unhappy way to live. Choosing to connect with others, however, opens us to the abundance of Love.

Give Love to Receive Love: The Circle of Connection

We make a living by what we get.
We make a life by what we give.
—Winston Churchill

At the most basic level, we all want to feel safe, accepted, and cared for. Many of us spend our entire lives in a headlong search for these basics, only to fail again and again. Why? Could it be that we crave Love and care, but are reluctant to give it? If so, our reluctance blocks the flow of Loving Energy for all of us.

Have you ever thought of calling someone and then you put it off? Love's voice might say, *You should call______. They could use a little love.* But then our self-centered thoughts close our hearts and whisper, *You don't have time. They don't really need your call.* Next, the fearful excuses pile up: *You might disturb them. Why would they want to talk to you, anyway?*

What's up with that? Why do I push back against Love's voice? Somewhere deep inside, I'm unwilling to care for that person, perhaps based on something they did or didn't do. Maybe they remind me of a painful situation, and my fear-filled thoughts distract me from acting. Or I might simply not want to make the effort.

When we allow our hearts to close in these ways, we separate ourselves from loving oneness and connection.

In contrast, when we reach out with open-hearted Love for others, they can offer it to another, who then opens their heart to another, and so on. It's a beautiful chain of infinite light that only grows when we give it to others.

This lesson from the nonprofit organization Attitudinal Healing expresses this truth so well: "We can become love finders rather than fault finders."[39] When we find fault, we criticize others in the arrogant belief that we know better, thus casting them out of our hearts and closing ourselves off from Loving Energy. Unfortunately, such destructive thoughts only make things worse, in our own minds and the world.

How, then, do we become Love finders? We connect our hearts with others via positive thoughts, prayers, and spoken words of hope, care, and affection. We choose to see the bright, True Self in each person, regardless of their words and actions. We get out of the judge's seat and leave that role to a power much wiser than we are. And we spread only Love, welcoming all—including ourselves—into the circle of belonging.

From now on, try to become a Love finder. Perhaps give a big smile to the checkout person at the grocery store and ask how their day is going. Or let someone into a line of traffic ahead of you. Maybe silently connect with the heart of a troubled person by thinking, *The light in me salutes the light in you.*

Trust me, you can have more harmonious open-hearted relationships when you awaken to your True Self and let its power take the lead. Begin with a willingness to let go of the blockages to Love. Continue with ongoing efforts to heal your resentments and fears. And then the fun part—top it off with loving acts of kindness toward everyone you meet.

Summary

- Holding on to resentments and criticism ruins our most important relationships.
- Every minute, we choose to either separate from or open our hearts to others.
- Resentment, self-deception, self-centered motives, and self-condemnation close our hearts, forming barriers to Love.
- Forgiveness is letting go of the ways we close our hearts to ourselves and others.
- The more we give Love to others, the more it comes back to fill our hearts.

For Your Consideration

These questions and statements invite you to apply this chapter's ideas to your life. As you reflect on them, consider adding questions of your own.

1. Who do you have a conflict with now? Why?
2. Try to feel loving compassion for yourself as you feel this pain. Observe it and know it is just part of being human.
3. What could your life be like without the pain of this conflict?
4. What patterns or fears are blocking your heart and contributing to conflict in your life?
5. What strategies will you use to help open your heart in this situation?

CHAPTER 5

Overcoming Life's Difficulties with an Open Heart

Worry not, my child.
You've elected to learn these lessons so that you can be free.
Walking through your worst fear transforms
it into an old meaningless fear.
Then a new worst fear will come to take its place.
Call the fear poverty, rejection, abandonment,
loneliness, death, meaninglessness, or helplessness.
What you forget is that you don't have
to walk through them alone.
We are simply rendering the barriers to love harmless
by walking through them together.

—Source unknown

Even though we've learned to connect with our True Selves, it doesn't mean we'll be smiling with bliss every minute of every day. Not at all! At any time, some event may throw us into a fearful, closed-hearted place of darkness, without apparent hope. As my first sponsor, Beth, says, "Life's in session."

I've had my share of life difficulties, and I'm sure you have, too. When faced with life's worries and disasters, we often fear they'll last forever, with nothing but pain and suffering ahead. In the quote above, however, we see that troublesome events can signal the beginning of significant learning—true growth in wisdom—if we stay awake and commit to opening our hearts. In short, we can harvest strength and wisdom from difficulty.

Every trial can be an opportunity to walk through our worst fear so it can become an old meaningless fear. With the Loving Energy of wise friends at our side, we move away from fear's whispered lies to the solutions offered by our loving True Selves. In turn, we're encouraged to embrace open-hearted living even more fully.

Remember, it's a process. We have to grow through several life challenges before we embrace them as lessons on the road to finding greater Love, joy, connection, and peace of mind.

First, we'll discuss a general process for working through troubling situations: the four Rs of Refrain, Reflect, Release, and Respond. Then, let's examine how to open our hearts to find wisdom and guidance when we're…

- worried about loved ones,
- concerned about our own illness and/or aging,
- stressed about work and creative pursuits, or
- disturbed about political conflict and world events.

I won't say it's easy to go through these difficulties with an open heart, but I *will* say it's worth it. As I face each one, I can remember how my True Self unerringly guided me through the last one—rendering the barriers to Love harmless.

The Four Rs: Refrain, Reflect, Release, Respond

We tend to believe our problems are causing our unwanted behaviors. It is only upon inspection that we learn the reverse to be true. It is most likely that our reactions to life are causing our problems.

—Freddie van Rensburg[40]

When a negative or scary thing happens to me or my loved ones, I often revert to feeling separate and alone, as depicted in the image of Closed-Hearted Separation on page 82. For example, when my niece's boyfriend confronted me about my plan for replacing my car battery, my heart closed, and I felt like a terrified, helpless child. In this fearful state, I lashed out at him. Afterward, I ended up painted into a corner of shame, feeling isolated and unlovable.

Fortunately, I don't have to stay in such hopelessness because my True Self beckons me to wake up to the truth. Perhaps it's a heart-stopping image of beauty, or the loving hand of a friend. In this golden moment, I begin to do the work to reopen my heart to Loving Energy and reconnect with my solid-on-the-inside wisdom.

But how do I do that, especially when fear is frantically tugging at me? I use the four Rs. First, I Refrain from acting; next, I Reflect on my part in the difficulty; then I marshal Loving Energy to Release the negativity blocking my heart. Finally, from the calm wisdom of my True Self, I Respond with actions I hope will benefit all involved.

My friend Erica used these four strategies to prepare for a potentially scary visit with her family for Thanksgiving dinner. Since her parents were elderly and lived 150 miles away, she always felt obliged to spend the night. But every time she went to a family dinner, her brothers got drunk and began arguing with her parents about politics. In the past, she had joined in the drinking and the arguments, always returning home resentful and disturbed.

But this year was different. Erica was in early recovery from her drinking problem and knew staying sober was a priority. She shared her confusion with me by saying, "I'm afraid they won't love me if I don't go; but I also don't want to put myself in such a threatening situation. I'm all mixed up!"

Refrain from Taking Direct Action

As mentioned in Chapter 4, when faced with a life challenge, our best action is to wait (Refrain). Another way to put it is to Postpone Action Until Serenity Emerges (PAUSE). From a place of serenity, we'll know how best to respond. But it isn't so easy to hit that pause button, right?

Instead, we often try for a quick fix, just so our icky feelings will go away. With adrenaline surging, we send that text or email or pick up the phone, just to help us feel better now. In most cases, however, acting too soon produces harmful words and actions that we never intended.

Fortunately, Erica had learned to hit the pause button before responding to any disturbing situation. So, when her mother called to invite her to Thanksgiving dinner, she said she needed some time to figure out how long she could stay.

During this pause, we refrain from punishing ourselves for being confused and instead practice self-compassion by remembering we're simply imperfect human beings doing the best we can. Such self-talk might sound like this: *Yes, this is hard, and I'm upset. But anyone in my position would find this difficult. I've got my loving True Self and others to help me figure this out.*

Reflect on Our Part in the Situation

The next step during the pause is to Reflect on our part in the situation by asking, *What is it about me that makes this so difficult?*

The following questions help us examine how we might be contributing to our unease. As you'll notice, they are derived from the six negative patterns described on page 38–40, and the four barriers to Love on page 85. Here is each question with Erica's response.

Six Negative Patterns from Chapter 3

1. **Caretaker**. How have I been putting others' needs above my self-care? *I have been trying to take care of my family's feelings by doing whatever would make them feel good. But I didn't take care of myself. I had it backward.*

2. **Martyr**. Do I sometimes feel like a victim of circumstances beyond my control? *Yes. I've felt stuck with no way out of this Thanksgiving dinner.*

3. **Perfectionist**. How have I been expecting myself and others to never make mistakes? *I'm afraid I won't make the perfect decision. I certainly have expected my brothers to be perfect, and to not get into political arguments with my parents. But they still do it.*

4. **People Pleaser**. How have I been pretending to be what others want me to be? *I never said a word to them about their behavior and how it affects me. I'm afraid they'll abandon me if I don't do what they want.*

5. **Workaholic**. How have I been placing work above my relationships and health? *Not applicable.*

6. **Tap Dancer.** How have I been unwilling to fully commit to my growth and healing? *I left any situation that got uncomfortable, thus depriving myself of the opportunity to grow through it. Now, I am finally so committed to my sobriety that I am willing to risk disappointing my parents.*

Four Barriers to Love from Chapter 4

1. **Resentment**. What person or circumstance am I resenting, blaming, or criticizing? What do I think they're "depriving" me of? *I criticized my parents for joining in with my brothers' political battles. I hated them all for getting drunk and ruining my enjoyment of the holiday dinner.*

2. **Self-Centered Motives.** Where have I been self-centered, thinking only of getting my needs met? *When I drank, I only thought about myself. I never reached out to visit them.*

3. **Self-Deception.** How have I been dishonest with myself or others? *I had been telling myself that family dinners would be different this time, that maybe they'd change. But every year I returned home with the same knot in my stomach.*

4. **Self-Condemnation.** What self-critical beliefs have I held about myself? *I thought there must be something wrong with me. It seemed like everyone else could handle these situations and I just couldn't.*

After answering the ten questions, it's helpful to select two of them, usually the ones that are causing the most distress, for further reflection. Then we dig a little deeper into how our needs, consequences, and desires relate to the issue. Here's how Erica reflected on her Caretaker pattern and her Resentments.

Caretaker: Deeper Reflection

a. What was I trying to gain by holding on to my Caretaking? *I was trying to gain emotional security, thinking if I put their needs before mine, they'd love me more.*

b. What are the negative consequences for me and others of holding on to this Caretaking behavior? *I might not stay sober if I don't put my own needs first.*

c. What could my life be like if I let go of my Caretaking? *I wouldn't rely on my family to help me feel secure and loved. I am learning my security comes only from Loving Energy and my recovery partners.*

Resentment: Deeper Reflection

a. What was I trying to gain by holding on to this Resentment? *The more I criticized them, the less I had to look at my own drinking.*

b. What are the negative consequences for me and others of holding on to this Resentment? *My anger might come out against my parents and damage my relationship with them. Also, if I don't resolve it, I may drink again.*

c. What could my life be like if I let go of this Resentment? *I could go to family dinners without fearing conflict. I would give myself permission to go only for as long as it feels safe. I could see the best in my family, rather than focusing on their faults.*

As you work through these ten questions for your own situation, please celebrate yourself for having the courage to face and release your limiting patterns and fears. Filling your heart with Loving Energy will animate your True Self, which leads you to the best solutions for all.

Release Negative Patterns and Barriers to Love

After sharing her reflections with me, Erica realized she needed to change, and could only do so with the power and wisdom of her True Self and her healthy friends. Together, we created this affirmation: "I release my negative patterns and fears concerning my family, and I see them with love, compassion, and patience."

Next, she visualized how she would like to feel and act in the future: "I have courage, compassion, and grace in my family interactions. I ensure my own safety and comfort in the best way for all involved."

Erica then wrote a plan of action to open her heart to solutions: "I constantly connect with the wisdom of my True Self. Every day I commit to saying and visualizing my affirmation, and using thought-switching, prayer, and guided meditations. I also read inspiring texts such as *The Four Agreements*[41] and *The Power of Now*[42] to dissolve my fears."

After several weeks of practicing these techniques, Erica said to me, "I don't want to keep hurting myself by hoping my family will change. I choose to accept them as they are. The good news is that I've found a new 'family' in recovery that loves me just the way I am."

Respond (Take Action) From a Place of Wisdom and Serenity

Remember Postpone Action Until Serenity Emerges (PAUSE)? Well, the time has come for action! After we've Refrained, Reflected, and Released, we've reconnected with the peace and wisdom in our True Selves. As a result, we find ourselves perceiving the troubling situation differently. Sometimes this happens quickly. Sometimes it's slower than molasses.

At some point, however, we find ourselves no longer blaming others for their part in our misery. And here's the bonus: We're able to take loving, assertive action without fear of reprisals because we know our True Self has our back.

Here's how Erica described her transformation and her response to her mother:

> "I now realize that none of my family members meant to hurt me; they were just acting out their old fear-driven patterns. But I don't have to engage in Caretaking anymore by putting their needs ahead of mine, especially if it isn't good for me. Also, I'm trying to see beyond my Resentment to the light of their True Selves, but that may take a while! If my family is unable to treat me well, I will spend less time there. I've decided to tell my mother that I will attend the Thanksgiving

> dinner, but I'll be driving home afterwards. Also, I've promised myself that if I feel uncomfortable at any time, I can go to the bathroom and call my sponsor or another supportive friend. I can even give myself permission to leave."

Now, on to considering four major life difficulties and how to address them with open-hearted wisdom.

Life Difficulty: Worry about Loved Ones

It seems natural to expect an outcome from my actions. The problem is that I have no control over the people that my actions involve, so when I expect a particular outcome, I am usually disappointed.

—Buddy C.

Opening our hearts to truly love a child, spouse, sibling, partner, friend, or parent is one of life's most wonderful experiences. However, if this care becomes an obsession about the safety of our loved ones, it can easily sabotage both our own serenity and the relationships we so cherish.

The difficulty often begins when we observe a loved one acting in dangerous ways. Perhaps it's a child whose use of alcohol or other drugs is threatening their life. It might show up as a spouse who, despite a recent heart attack, refuses to eat healthy foods or exercise. Or it could be a sister falling in love with an abusive man. Observing these situations, our fear whispers, *What will I do if they are hurt or die? How will I possibly cope with it? I don't think I can live without them. I must do something to stop it!*

We wouldn't be human if we didn't have such fears, right? At first, they scare the pants off us, closing our hearts to the wisdom of our True Selves. Disconnected from this guidance and feeling alone, we try to prevent the impending disaster the only way our fear allows, by desperately trying to control the other person.

It never works. When they fail to take our advice, it worries us even more. We go into a tailspin of anxiety as we keep trying to force change on them, succeeding only in pushing them farther away.

Many label this pattern as *codependency*, doing everything you can to remove the pain or dysfunction from your loved one without regard to your well-being. People caught in this trap see themselves as Martyrs *(If only he would change, I could be happy)*, Caretakers *(I have to take care of him all the time because nobody else will)*, or plain old "control freaks."

Even more troubling, codependents locate their happiness not within themselves, but within the other person's well-being. Therefore, they're content only when their loved one isn't drinking, overeating, using drugs, ill, overworking, or depressed. But when that person reverts to the disturbing state, the codependent's serenity evaporates. Quite often, they fall prey to exhaustion, depression, bitterness, or a variety of other ailments.

This story about my friend Nancy and her daughter illustrates how Al-Anon Family Groups can help loved ones of alcoholics and addicts overcome their misery. Since codependency is a form of addiction, Al-Anon follows the same Twelve Steps as AA. (See Chapter 6 for more information about the Twelve Steps and other addictions.)

Nancy was at her wit's end when her daughter, Wanda, returned to using alcohol and drugs after her third stay at a rehab treatment center. Wanda was nineteen and felt she could live her life as she wanted, despite the emotional and financial burdens on her parents.

Nancy and her husband, Pablo, had tried everything to save Wanda. They paid for apartments, relocations, and rehabs. But nothing helped. Wanda just kept latching onto addicted men and relapsing. Finally, they consulted a therapist who suggested they attend at least six Al-Anon meetings before deciding if they could be helpful.

In Al-Anon, Nancy and Pablo found parents and spouses of alcoholics who had been just as desperate as they. As group members shared how they found serenity, in spite of their loved ones' alcohol problems, Nancy and Pablo began to have hope. Soon, they each asked a sponsor to help them work the Twelve Steps to gain freedom from their constant worry.

Since the next chapter contains extensive detail about the Twelve Steps, here I'll stick with the four Rs to illustrate how Nancy and Pablo opened their hearts to gain courage and wisdom.

- *Refrain.* Nancy and Pablo honestly admitted their daughter's problem was hurting their health and marriage, and that they couldn't fix it on their own. In therapy and meetings, they recognized they could access a Loving Energy greater than their fears, and that sometimes this wisdom would come through their sponsor, therapist, or people at meetings. In the meantime, they would not take any actions to influence their daughter's behavior.

- *Reflect.* Nancy and Pablo examined their part in their worries and shared their insights with their sponsor. First, they admitted they were terrified of losing their daughter, and that they'd been Self-Deceptive by thinking their efforts would fix the problem. They also realized they were trying to reduce their fears by Caretaking; for example, by finding Wanda new lodgings and paying for her groceries. Finally, they were engaging in constant Self-Condemnation because they felt so helpless and ineffective.

- *Release*. Nancy and Pablo practiced connecting with the Loving Energy of their True Selves to dissolve the harmful aspects they'd discovered. For example, Nancy used prayer, while Pablo preferred meditation. They opened themselves to compassion for themselves and received valuable guidance from their sponsor and therapist.
- *Respond (Take Action)*. They began to put their daughter's future in Love's hands and set strict limits on how they would provide financial support; for example, only upon proof of attending a structured recovery program. Soon, they found themselves feeling less worried and taking better care of their own needs. As they continued their growth, they began helping other Al-Anon members find peace of mind, no matter what their loved ones were doing.

Nancy and Pablo report that Wanda is now thriving in a new rehab program and seems to be on the right track. To keep their boundaries and maintain their serenity, they still attend Al-Anon meetings.

As you've been reading about Nancy's dilemma, you might have noticed that Al-Anon can be helpful for any relationship challenge; for example, with May's abusive ex-husband and his family, and Paula's struggle with her step-daughter, Lisa. I have worked Al-Anon extensively and have found it to be extremely helpful, especially when my dear friend relapsed and almost died.

Even though we certainly don't have the power to change our loved ones, when we adjust our own attitudes and responses, the people around us often begin to mysteriously transform. After all, we're connected in our hearts. But even if our loved ones don't change for the better, we've found the peace of mind to allow them their consequences. Plus, we have a new courage, grace, and compassion toward ourselves.

Life Difficulty: Illness and Aging

We who have lived in our bodies for so many years, savoring its sensations, have made it the source of such joy. Now we ponder a single rude fact: clearly it was never meant to last. Without this body, though, what remains? Perhaps we've seen glimmers of it all along, a pure, sweet light, shared and amplified. As we witness our beloved bodies deteriorate, we know with tear-filled certainty: There was only ever this light, this love.

—Gigi Langer

I've had a lot of physical pain in my lifetime, and I've hated it. Doesn't everyone? But we know we can't avoid it. A tooth will decay, a joint will stiffen, or an accident may occur.

There are unlimited possibilities. Honestly, sometimes it's amazing that we even venture out of our homes!

When younger, I was a jock. I played tennis with the guys, rode horses over five-foot hurdles, and skied competitively. I thought I was indestructible. In the first year after I quit drinking, however, I badly sprained my ankle and, a few months later, had major abdominal surgery. Then I injured my back and suffered with that pain for years. In my mid-forties, I had frozen shoulders, which caused limited mobility for two years. It was impossible to wash my hair, and I could barely turn my car's steering wheel. My shoulders' flexibility returned only after two surgeries.

Looking back, I can see how these torturous problems taught me the importance of opening my heart to Love. First, they slowed down my Workaholism. I had been so used to rushing around that perhaps I needed to be stopped short (again and again) until I could learn to care for myself.

Most importantly, however, the physical pain helped me admit how powerless I was over my body. For years, I thought that if I could analyze the sources of pain, exercise properly, and avoid the wrong activities, I'd be able to ward off pain and illness. But such preoccupations only kept me stuck in thoughts of suffering and distress.

When I finally acknowledged that constant worrying about my physical problems was keeping me tense and unhappy, just the right resource turned up (prompted by

Loving Energy, no doubt). One day, a friend suggested I listen to a CD by Pema Chödrön,[43] a highly revered American Buddhist nun. Her suggestion to sit alongside my pain, observing it with patience and self-compassion, led me to my current meditation practice (MBSR)[44] one of my best antidotes to pain.

Another gift from those years of discomfort was learning to ask for help. Until getting sober, I had been fiercely independent, needing no one but my current man and perhaps one other friend. I thought I was an island and could handle anything that came my way. But, in recovery from alcoholism and my many illnesses, I gave up my rigid independence and admitted that I needed help; that I couldn't do it all by myself.

I believe I've finally come to terms with my body's frailties, but now I'm facing the challenge of aging. As health concerns mount up with my husband, siblings, and loved ones, I've had to look death squarely in the eye and face the age-old question: *Is my body all there is of me?*

Although none of us knows for sure, I choose to believe the *ACIM* lesson "I am not a body; I am free as Love created me."[45] It reminds me that my True Self has no need for a body, as it is beyond this place and time.

Unfortunately, we are exceedingly attached to our own and others' bodies, believing that what we do with them (travel, sports, and enjoying material things), brings us happiness. Not so! I bet you realize, as I do, that our greatest joy does not come from simple physical pleasures such as food or luxurious dwellings.

If you're on board with open-hearted living, you probably realize that the highest use of our bodies is to express loving care. For example, when we speak and hear loving words, hold hands with a grieving friend, or hug a child, we cultivate lasting peace and happiness.

Regardless of how we think about what happens to us after death, one thing is for sure: We're happiest when we connect with Love in the present moment. So, let's open our hearts and savor life, both the physical and the spiritual, regardless of the condition of our body.

Life Difficulty: Work and Creative Pursuits

Our fears, whether large or small, were distorted. And we still distort those fears, on occasion, because we move away from the spiritual reality of our lives.

—Karen Casey

Many daunting life difficulties arise when we are trying to accomplish a big project. It could be for school, work, or on our own time. We feel called to do it, flattered even, but then the whispered lies raise their ugly heads. The project seems to take forever, technology doesn't work, we get stuck in procrastination, or we lose courage altogether. In short, our hearts close up with fear, and we begin to lose our way. Here we consider how to overcome perfectionism, lack of motivation, and procrastination.

Perfectionism: A Way Through

Recently, I taught a workshop on how to overcome worry. During the session, I felt rushed and tense, possibly because I had planned too many things for the seventy-five minutes. In my agitation, I made a few mistakes. I forgot to do the prayer at the beginning, and during our Master Mind activity, I forgot two crucial steps. To my chagrin, a participant had to remind me to add them.

Although I laughed about it at the time, later my old pattern of Perfectionism grabbed my mental microphone and insisted I had embarrassed myself. In a panic, I then tried to figure out why I had made the mistakes, clinging to the false hope that I would never do so again. This self-punishment and constant analysis of my errors exhausted me, subtly draining my enthusiasm over the next few days.

Eventually, I acknowledged the cloud over my head and my true self nudged me: *We need some time to get our head straight.* The next day, I cleared my calendar, had coffee with my husband, and then lay down for a healing session with Loving Energy.

First, my kitty came and cuddled up on my tummy. (How does she know just when to appear?) I relaxed my body and breathed slowly as I imagined angels surrounding me. As I asked for help, their loving presence soothed my jagged feelings.

Then something surprising happened: I felt several dark strands of self-defeating beliefs being lifted out of my body. Even the whispered lie, *I can't be loved unless I am perfect*, floated away into a haze of Love. And there I lay, free to trust Love's wisdom to guide my efforts.

After a few more moments, I had an inspired thought. Since I had planned to talk about Byron Katie's *The Work* at the next session, I realized I could illustrate its use with my whispered lie, *I should not make mistakes*. I immediately got up and wrote out my answers to Katie's four questions, and then played with a few of her "turnarounds," where we look at the opposite of each belief. You can see the example I used with my class on page 123.

After doing the two turnarounds, I could feel my whispered lie, *I should not make mistakes,* shifting and my perspective changing. Afterward, I drew these conclusions.

- By believing I must be perfect, I was closing my heart to myself and opening the door to Self-Condemnation.
- Holding others to my perfectionistic standards caused me to feel judgmental and critical of them, thus separating me from Love.

- By releasing my whispered lie, Love flowed back into my heart, restoring my connection with my True Self and others.

I am so glad Loving Energy helped me shed another layer of Perfectionism that had been blocking my True Self. But most of all, I'm grateful that my True Self inspired me to write this, share it with my class, and include it in this book.

Byron Katie's Four Questions with Two Turnarounds[46]

False belief: ***I should not make mistakes.***

1. Is it true? *Yes, I've always thought so.*
2. Is it completely true? *No, there might be good reasons for making mistakes.*
3. What's the emotional cost of this belief? *My loss of sleep and achy neck.*
4. What could my life be like without this belief? *I could relax in loving acceptance of myself when I make mistakes. I could open my heart to myself and others.*

Turnaround #1 (change a positive or negative word to its opposite): *I should not make mistakes* becomes ***I should (be able to) make mistakes.***
Is this turnaround statement truer than the first one? *Yes, because it's okay for me to make mistakes. I'm only human, and my mistakes have nothing to do with my security or worth. It could also be true because it creates a serendipitous teaching opportunity for my class by illustrating how I got hung up by my old negative patterns. So, perhaps my mistakes can be a good thing!*

Turnaround #2 (change the subject of sentence): ***They should not make mistakes.***
Is this turnaround statement truer than the first one? *No. It's not true at all. It's okay for others to make mistakes.*

Finding Motivation for Creative and Work Projects

It's easy to sabotage a creative project despite our passion for it. The cherished dream calls to us, but every time we think about working on it, we find tons of reasons not to. In the back of our minds, a chorus of whispered lies tells us that we're not capable of rising to this challenge.

I had this discouraging experience after an editor and some other readers suggested major changes to the first draft of *50 Ways to Worry Less Now*. I could hear fear whispering, *What if the changes ruin it? How could I possibly do that much rewriting? Will it ever be good enough?* Suddenly, my progress came to a halt.

Even though I knew there was a way forward, I couldn't yet see it. After years of practice, I knew enough to connect with my True Self through continuing my meditations and affirmations. I waited and continued going to meetings, doing service work, and using other growth tools. A few days later, I ran across a blog by Steven Pressfield explaining how to break through blocks to creativity by using these four questions from *The War of Art*.[47] Here are my responses to these thought-provoking questions.

1. What painful ideas are keeping me from finishing my book?
    - *If I spend so much time writing, I'll miss out on lots of fun.*

- *It might not be good enough; perhaps I've wasted my time.*
- *I dread the publishing process and the marketing after I finish.*

2. What pleasure can be gained from finishing it?
   - *I love teaching about ways to replace worry with kindness and Love.*
   - *I could find out how the book has helped others.*
   - *I would feel grateful to Loving Energy for helping me get it done.*

3. What will it cost me if I don't complete it?
   - *I'd feel embarrassed because a lot of people know about it.*
   - *I would let down the part of me that's inspiring me to do this.*
   - *I would continue to be jealous of other successful authors.*

4. Why is completing my book so important?
   - *I want others to use the concepts and tools to be free of worry and fear so they can be loving, happy, and content.*

- *It shares who I am with readers so they can be inspired to grow through their difficult times, just as I have.*
- *It's a useful resource because it's a compendium of many helpful tools.*

The answers to these questions reignited my motivation and I got back to work. Within a year, I had an advance copy ready for reviewers. In February 2018, I released the completed book. Finding myself at my first book signing event, I gasped in amazement. I was experiencing exactly what I had visualized for so many years! My dream had come true.

Tips for Overcoming Procrastination

Procrastination is the kidnapper of souls and the recruiting-officer of hell.

—Edward Irving

I've had a lot of experience with procrastination and have found a few techniques that help me get even the most challenging tasks done. The first one involves writing lists, where the page becomes the container for my free-floating "shoulds" and anxieties. List-making also counters the irrational belief that I must remember everything I need to do. I hope these ideas work for you, too.

- Make a master list of all the things you both want and need to get done in the near future. Breathe and tell yourself that you do not have to get them all done today.
- Put a star next to the ones that must be done today. For example, "Order paper" or "Shop for food."
- Write the starred items on a new list called To-Do Today. Now it doesn't look so long and overwhelming, right?
- On the master list, circle the important-but-not-urgent items, those that will ultimately improve your life or work. For example, "Exercise," or "Meet with (an emotionally healthy friend)" or "Write proposal."
- Write the circled items on a new list called "Important" and schedule them in your calendar. If you don't get to a particular item that day, move it to another day. But don't delete it.
- Get started on your To-Do Today list.

    1. Pick one easy thing to do first. Do that one thing and pat yourself on the back. Then go get a cup of coffee or tea. Smile!

    2. Return to your workspace and look at the item you just crossed off. Breathe in a good

feeling about doing that one thing. Do not think about the rest of the list.

3. Select another item and proceed as in Steps 1 and 2.

4. If you get tense, worried, or resistant, go somewhere private. Take a few belly-inflating breaths and loosen your jaw and shoulders. Tell yourself, *How I'm feeling right now is okay. If I do one thing at a time, what's necessary will get done.* Then go back to your list and complete an easy item.

5. Keep working your way through the list, taking short breaks, and patting yourself on the back. If necessary, re-evaluate the list and move the less-urgent items to another day.

On my own To-Do Today list, I wrote "Create one new social media ad." On my Important list, I put making a video, recording an audiobook, and scheduling a speaking engagement. Although I know I don't need to do all of the important items right away, I put reminders in my calendar so I don't forget them.

Here's a second powerful hack for overcoming procrastination. Set a timer for fifteen minutes and tell yourself you can stop working when it rings. If you feel like continuing, set the timer for another fifteen minutes. This takes you off the hook of thinking that the only success is finishing the entire task.

I know you can achieve the dreams that may now seem unreachable. The more you open your heart, connect with Love, and join with other inspiring people, however, the easier it will be to access your creative energy and fulfill your destiny.

Life Difficulty: Political Conflict and World Events

Three years ago, I made the mistake of posting something political on Facebook. I awoke to a tirade of anger from a few of my dearest friends and panicked when I thought I had lost them. I was tempted to respond with a fiery comment but knew I needed to refrain for the time being.

For many years, I had felt shame and fear around political talk and knew it was a tender area for me. So, I sat with my feelings and honestly admitted that I was really upset. After a while, I realized I needed to invite Loving Energy into my troubled mind. I said a prayer and asked to see my friends' reactions differently.

I knew I had an important choice to make. I could either consider my friends' responses as a personal attack or I could use the opportunity to heal my hot feelings toward this imagined offense. This would require some serious reflection.

First, I pondered these questions: *When did I first feel these feelings? Are they still valid?* I always know I hit pay dirt when the tears come. In this case, I recalled my mom spending many hours talking on the phone about politics. Her loud, angry tone always terrified me. But mostly I longed for her to put down the phone and give me her attention. She rarely did.

When I read my friends' testy responses to my Facebook post, I felt just like that little girl, afraid of my mom's politically fueled anger. My whispered lies told me, *Stay away from politics. It can only hurt you.* Recognizing this familiar fear, I was able to reassure my inner child that we weren't facing my mother's anger. *I'm here, and you are loved. None of this can hurt you.*

As the day progressed, I kept worrying about my friends' attitudes toward me. To restore my peace of mind, I used thought-switching to affirm, *I see only peace instead of conflict.* Gradually, my True Self reminded me that there was no need to separate from my friends because of their responses. That afternoon, I removed my post. I never needed to mention it to my friends, because it wasn't about them; it was only about my fear-filled reactions.

Imagining personal attacks from others causes us to close our hearts to them. When we recognize that fear is the source of these feelings and connect with Love instead, we find that nothing can separate us from our friends' hearts, not even politics.

Now let's move on to scary world events. It's pretty easy to get disturbed when the world appears to be falling apart. For example, when we tune into our favorite cable news shows, fear and judgment can overwhelm us. Sadly, what we see in the media often presses the panic button in our psyches.

I'm not suggesting that we avoid all media and bury our heads in the sand. Not so. I read a variety of news articles. I also write to my local and national representatives and, of course, I vote. But I try my best to refrain from judging others because of their beliefs or how they express them.

My approach to the daily news is partially summarized in this phrase, "The best attitude to cultivate is gentle indifference."[48] I think of indifference as detachment—a way of standing apart without getting caught up in the drama of arguments, while still acting from the peace and integrity of our True Selves.

Here's how I try to detach from scary thoughts about the world so I can remain open to Love.

- The minute I hear troubling news, I pray for those involved, that they may be guided to the best solutions for all involved.
- When I'm tempted to respond negatively, I take a few deep breaths and affirm that everything is

in perfect order, even if my fear-filled perceptions tell me it's not.

- I trust that by opening my heart, I will be guided to the right thoughts, words, and actions.
- I accept that my goal is to be a channel of Love, not fear.
- As a highly sensitive person, I limit my exposure to inflammatory news sources.

Finally, here's some good advice on media consumption from the Franciscan priest and spiritual writer, Richard Rohr.

> "I recommend for your spiritual practice for the next four months that you ***impose a moratorium on exactly how much news you are subject to***—hopefully not more than an hour a day of television, social media, internet news, magazine and newspaper commentary, and/or political discussions. Use this time for some form of public service, volunteerism, mystical reading from the masters, prayer—or, preferably, all of the above. You have much to gain now and nothing to lose. Nothing at all. And the world—with you as a stable center—has nothing to lose. And everything to gain."[49]

When I follow Rohr's advice, I'm far more peaceful and loving toward others because I'm not riled up by fears about events I can't control. And I focus on what I can control: my thoughts and actions as a citizen of this country.

Although the life difficulties discussed above are common, another obstacle to health and peace affects a surprising number of us: alcoholism and other addictions. In fact, over 10 percent of the U.S. population struggles with substance use. Given the extent of the problem, I've dedicated the next chapter to it.

Summary

- We can successfully face life's difficulties by refraining from immediate action, reflecting on our part in the dilemma, releasing our negativity, and responding with actions guided by our serene True Selves.
- Worrying about the safety of loved ones can harm us and them. We can overcome codependency with Al-Anon or other programs to help us detach with Love.
- Illness and aging are significant challenges for many of us. It helps to know our True Selves are not bound to our body and will likely go on as Loving Energy.
- Work and creative pursuits often trigger perfectionism, lack of motivation, and procrastination.

We relieve these blocks to Love's expression through growth tools and connecting with others.

- Political conflict and world events can spur fear and division among us. We strive for an open, tolerant, and kind approach as we find the right balance for our serenity.

For Your Consideration

As you ponder the following questions, go back to your responses after the preface, page xxiiv. What growth are you noticing in how you're dealing with your life difficulties? Again, you may choose to write or draw your responses.

1. Which situations in your life might require you to refrain from acting until you can find peace of mind?

2. As you have reflected on your part in a troubling situation, what have you learned about yourself?

3. Which tools and practices have helped you release old self-defeating patterns?

4. Of the four life difficulties mentioned here, which one or two are ongoing concerns for you?

5. What ideas and tools might help you connect with the wisdom of your True Self to find new ways of responding to your challenges?

CHAPTER 6

Opening Our Hearts after Addiction

Addiction is like a cancer that overpowers
and destroys its host.
—Bohunk

I am closing *Love More Now* with this chapter because I believe that alcoholism and other addictions are the ultimate heart closers. When fear whispers, *I can't stand feeling this way. I must numb myself to get relief*, the person has lost the ability to access the True Self's hope, trust, and peace of mind.

As expressed in AA literature, they are cut off from "the sunlight of the spirit,"[50] or what we've been referring to as Loving Energy or True Self. Such barren loneliness is the hallmark of the disease of addiction.

Many erroneously believe that people choose to be addicted, and therefore, it's a personal failure: *If they only tried harder, they could overcome it.* But this is far from the truth. The official medical opinion is that addictions are caused by a genetic predisposition and social factors.[51] Most important, the disease is considered a brain disorder as serious as any neurological or mental illness.[52]

Addictions include the use of alcohol, illegal drugs, food, and prescribed drugs (not just opiates, but any pill that immediately soothes our emotions). Gambling, shopping, and sex can also become addictive. Although the addicted person believes the habit helps them get through life's challenges, it ends up hurting more than helping. In the U.S. alone, one in five deaths among twenty- to forty-nine-year-olds were caused by alcohol consumption.[53]

What does addiction look like? It's a chronic, relapsing disorder characterized by the following:

- Compulsive behavior or compulsively seeking the drug, alcohol, other substances, or behavior.
- Preoccupation with the substance or behavior.
- Continued use despite harmful consequences.
- Gradual escalation until control is lost.
- Long-lasting changes in the brain.[54]

Do I Have a Problem?

Sometimes I wonder if addicts aren't all that different from anybody else, they are just better at lying to themselves.

—Taylor Jenkins Reid

Trust me, if your life isn't working, your relationships are awful, you grew up in a dysfunctional family, or you identify with the ways we close our hearts to ourselves, you're at risk for using addictive habits to find relief from your everyday troubles.

Please, don't let denial get in the way. Take a long look in the mirror. You're the only one who can do something about your problem. If you have two or more of the symptoms listed in this quiz, you probably need to see a doctor or therapist to begin recovering.

1. There is a desire to cut down on use or unsuccessful efforts to cut down.

2. The substance or activity is used in larger amounts, or for a longer period of time than was intended.

3. The pursuit of the substance or activity consumes a significant amount of time.

4. There is a craving—a strong desire—to use the substance or engage in the activity.

5. Use of the substance or activity disrupts obligations at work, school, or home.

6. Use of the substance or activity continues despite the serious problems it causes.

7. Participation in important social, work, or recreational activities drops or stops.

8. Use occurs in situations where it is physically risky.

9. Use continues despite knowing it is the source of escalating physical or psychological problems.

10. Tolerance occurs, indicated either by a need for a markedly increased amount of the substance to achieve the desired effect or markedly diminished effect of the same amount of substance.

11. Physiological withdrawal occurs, or a related substance is taken to block the discomfort.[55]

You might ask, *Why is this habit of mine a problem? Shouldn't we all be able to feel better as quickly as possible?* Not if we want to grow emotionally. Think of it this way: When we have unpleasant feelings, we have two choices—to numb them or to learn how to grow through them. The only way to awaken to your open-hearted True Self is to choose growth rather than denial.

When you do the work to recover your best self, you'll have no need to medicate your unwanted feelings away, no matter what is going on in your life.

Unfortunately, in our society, we face the belief that we can't have fun without alcohol or other drugs. It's in our faces every minute of every day, right? Partying is the main "fun" activity in our culture. Watching sports? Have a beer! Going out with friends? Have a few drinks! Unfortunately, the initial pleasure of a few drinks can accelerate into multiple drinks and drugs with no stopping point until we pass out, get arrested, or ruin our health.

Toward the end of our years of drinking, drugging, gambling, or another habit, we're often completely isolated, as our closed hearts have separated us from healthy, loving people. If we're lucky, we get the gift of desperation and begin to seek a new way of living.

Because my experience is with Alcoholics Anonymous (AA), and because of the recent Stanford research study[56] documenting its effectiveness, I focus here on how working the Twelve Steps opens our hearts to our True Selves. If you wish, you may substitute Loving Energy or True Self for AA's language of a higher power or God. But remember, it's your conception of a power greater than your troubles that will save your life. Don't let mere terminology stop you.

What Is AA? Do the Twelve Steps Work?

AA began in 1935 when two men in Akron, Ohio, were searching for a way to stay sober. They were able to do so by forming a support group and developing the Twelve Steps. The AA model, open to all and free, has spread around the globe, and AA now boasts over two million members in 180 nations and more than 118,000 groups.[57]

An extensive Stanford research review found AA to be more effective in promoting sobriety than other interventions or no intervention. One study found AA was 60 percent more effective, and another showed that AA and Twelve-Step counseling reduced mental health costs by $10,000 per person. The findings were consistent whether participants were young, elderly, male, female, veterans, civilians, or from outside the USA.[58]

The Twelve Steps have been applied to a variety of addictions. Groups exist for people struggling with codependency, overeating, gambling, narcotics, crystal meth, marijuana, self-injury, sex, emotions, and incest. Each group uses the same Twelve Steps from AA, but with a single change: In Step 1, the word "alcohol" is typically replaced with the name of the addiction treated. Finally, the only requirement for attending Twelve-Step meetings is the desire to stop your addiction(s).

We Can't Do It Alone

Don't try to kill your pain. Share it with another. When you lighten your burden and discover the jewels and joy alive beneath the pain, later you'll be present for others who are suffering.

—Cuong and Lu

As I've said time and time again, we can't change our lives all by ourselves. We need others who have gone before us, people who have learned to take life "uncut" with patience, tolerance, and courage. With understanding and help from others, we learn how to face our unpleasant feelings head-on, without the need to deny them.

I was a loner before I admitted my alcoholism, so I understand how difficult it can be to find such friends. If you're a loner too, I encourage you to be open-minded and keep searching for support. Even one emotionally healthy person is enough for now, perhaps a friend or therapist.

Connecting with recovering people helps in at least three ways. First, it's easier to be honest with yourself when you're around people who openly share their personal struggles and victories. As you listen, you can tune into your feelings and uncover some of your own whispered lies. Second, with such friends, you can find self-acceptance and hope that may elude you when you're alone. As others describe their lives before recovery, you begin to realize you're not the only one who has done horrible things, and that you too can overcome your problems.

Third, you'll often find subtle guidance through others. As people tell their stories, you might hear just the words you need. In turn, you may hear yourself saying things that are helpful not only to your sober friends but also to yourself. Finally, we have amazingly bad memories. For any new way of life to stick, we need constant reminders of the key principles and tools of recovery.

If you decide to attend Twelve-Step meetings regularly, you'll find the right recovering buddies, plus a sponsor to guide you through the Steps. Please just keep showing up. I still attend meetings and work the Steps today, even after more than thirty years of continuous sobriety. Why? Because they keep me connected with Love, and I get to see the most amazing personal transformations from a front-row seat.

How the Twelve Steps Open Our Hearts

Learning is invisible, and what has been learned can be recognized only by its results.

—ACIM

The Twelve Steps illustrate this quote beautifully, as seen in this brief overview.

- *Steps 1–3.* When we accept our personal powerlessness and start to trust a Loving Energy greater than our addiction, we begin to notice surprisingly visible changes in our lives: we're enjoying meetings; we're seeking out healthy, sober mentors and friends; and most important, we aren't practicing our addictive habits.

- *Steps 4–9.* As we take responsibility for and apply the program to our self-centered fears and actions, we gradually act more generously toward ourselves and others. In short, our invisible internal changes begin to manifest as positive outer changes.
- *Steps 10–12.* As we continue to replace fear, resentment, and worry with Love, trust, and connection, we share it with others.

Working the Twelve Steps changes us inside. And those changes show up as visible results, in living color. Observe anyone honestly working the Twelve Steps, and over time, you'll see them grow into their True Self: mature, calm, and capable of handling life's ups and downs without self-medicating. Further, you'll find them living from an open heart of generosity and care.

Here I translate The Twelve Steps of Alcoholics Anonymous into the language we've been using throughout this book. For each Step, I first list its main principle, and then the original language for that Step.

Step 1. Honesty

We admitted we were powerless over alcohol—that our lives had become unmanageable.

My favorite AA axiom is: "SOBER spells Son Of a Bitch, Everything's Real!" Hearing this phrase smashed my self-deception as I began to face and accept how crazy my life had become.

Interestingly, most people think their problems cause them to seek relief through their addiction. But it's the opposite: addiction is causing problems. Little growth can happen until we accept two things: we've been using a habit or substance to get through life, and we've not been able to stop using it. It's finally time to accept our part in causing our problems and do something about it.

Back in Chapter 1 on page 9, we saw the person with a closed heart and the person with an open heart. The one with a closed heart has allowed their worries, blame, and denial to restrict the flow of Love into their life. In the case of addiction, their preoccupation and dependence have hidden the gifts of their True Selves. They believe that deep down they are bad people, and nothing can be done to change that. No wonder they feel they have to drink or drug those feelings away.

Once we've accepted that we *do* have a problem and we can't fix it on our own, we come to Steps 2 and 3. We ask ourselves, *How might a higher power (Loving Energy or True Self) lead us in the right direction?*

Step 2. Hope

Came to believe that a Power greater than ourselves could restore us to sanity.

The key principle of Step 2 is HOPE, perhaps standing for Heart Open, Please Enter—an invitation to Loving Energy (and recovering people) to help us learn how to love.

In Chapter 1, we claimed that we can open our hearts to this Loving Energy, a force for goodness and healing. Further, we asserted that this Love is always available to us. But do we really believe it? In the early days of recovery, it can be a tough sell.

As we read Step 2 and grapple with our doubts about "a Power greater than ourselves," we don't let the word "believe" hang us up. It does not mean that we must be 100 percent certain that this power exists. No. We're merely *entertaining the idea* that there is something bigger and wiser than our own fearful thinking. And maybe tapping into this Loving Energy can restore us to a place of peace and happiness.

Just follow hope, open your heart, and say, *Please enter.* Even with the tiniest amount of belief, little shots of inspiration and intuition begin to seep into our minds. In Step 3, we make a decision to give this Love more influence over our lives.

Step 3. Faith

Made a decision to turn our will and our lives over to the care of God as we understood Him.

Since the principle of faith can turn people off, I often use the word *trust*. In fact, I have a long, wide ribbon hanging in my closet that says, "Trust Love." I created it long ago, when I had my first inkling that the Twelve Steps could work for me—even if I wasn't so sure about the God language.

Let's now consider what I think of as the most important word in Step 3: *care*. Please know it doesn't mean that we turn our will and lives over to the *control* of God, as many fear. No. We're deciding to turn our thoughts (our will) and actions (our lives) over to the *comforting care* and love of God. Only that.

Now notice the words, "God *as we understood Him*." We're invited to come to our conception of a power greater than our fears and problems. No one is asking us to believe a certain set of ideas about a higher power. In my case, my first concept was of a female divine energy. However we frame this loving power, it is our portal to a calm wisdom that intuitively knows how to handle any challenge that comes our way.

When we are ready to make the decision, we say this Step 3 prayer with our sponsor. Feel free to replace the *thees* and *thous*, and even the word *God*. But give it a sincere try. Open your heart and invite that Loving Energy in.

> "God, I offer myself to Thee—to build with me and to do with me as Thou wilt.
>
> Relieve me of the bondage of self, that I may better do Thy will.
>
> Take away my difficulties, that victory over them may bear witness to those I would help of Thy Power, Thy Love, and Thy Way of life.
>
> May I do Thy will always."[59]

First, we assert that we want to align ourselves with God's will. We might think of God's will as the goodness of Loving Energy, nudging us toward ever more just and caring actions.

Now, let's focus on the second sentence, "Relieve me of the bondage of self." What is the bondage of self? You've been reading about it throughout this book. It's the fear-driven, selfish part of you that is running amok, interested only in getting its own needs met, often to the detriment of others. This "me, myself, and I" thinks it has everything handled, but its closed-hearted selfishness keeps failing, especially in relationships. In essence, our self-centered thinking has been keeping our True Selves in bondage.

When we take Step 3, we declare to the universe that we are willing to change, to become less fearful and more open-hearted. That's a great start, but it's only a beginning. Next, we need to look at the exact nature of the patterns and barriers that have been blocking our hearts.

Step 4. Courage

Made a searching and fearless moral inventory of ourselves.

Notice the word *fearless.* You might ask, *Where do we get the courage to go on?* Note that *coeur,* the French word for heart, is the root word for courage. For some time now, you've been opening your heart to this powerful flow of Love. And now it's time to use it.

Let's face it, addiction is the opposite of courage. It's the chicken's way out. *I can't handle who I am, so I'll hide it.* Once into recovery, many balk at Step 4, as fear and shame whisper, *I don't want to face it. All that nasty stuff will come gushing out and overwhelm me.* When we're afraid to go on, many suggest backing up to the prior Step until we can trust that Love has our backs. It's also helpful to begin the inventory with a list of our assets.

Although I too feared that the ugly would come out all at once, that didn't happen. In fact, the wisdom of my True Self allowed my secrets to emerge only when I was ready. Some of the scariest things didn't arise until I was a few years sober, thank God!

So, how do we take a fearless moral inventory? The primary text of AA illustrates how to examine our resentments,

fears, and sexual behavior. In each area, we are to consider how we've been holding on to the four main barriers to Love discussed earlier: Resentment, Self-Centered Motives, Self-Deception, and Self-Condemnation.

As we move through the steps, we notice how certain roles learned early in life have been sabotaging our ability to function in healthy ways. I described these six patterns in Chapter 2, pages 38–40: Caretaker, Martyr, Perfectionist, People Pleaser, Workaholic, and Tap Dancer. In Chapter 4, pages 83–85, you'll see how I combined the four barriers and six patterns into a ten-question inventory that may be helpful in understanding how we've been contributing to our misery in the face of life's challenges.

By reflecting on our habitual responses in this way, we can begin to face and change them. But only if we don't keep them a secret.

Step 5. Integrity

Admitted to God, to ourselves, and to another human being the exact nature of our wrongs.

I've often heard that we're only as sick as our secrets. Indeed, what stays hidden tends to spawn shame and guilt, corrosive poisons that eat away at us. The purpose of Step 5 is to dissolve the shame that's been blocking the integrity of our True Selves.

When we share our inventory with our sponsor or a trusted third party, we're amazed that they don't frown or go running away when they hear our misdeeds. Often, they reply by sharing a few of their own, some of them quite awful. This caring experience goes a long way toward healing our self-condemning whispered lies. Remember the Master-Beaters Club in Chapter 2, page 29–30? That habit began to dissolve as I felt my sponsor's unwavering loving care, regardless of the secrets I revealed to her.

Although facing another human being with my flaws wasn't easy, the hardest part was admitting them to God (Loving Energy). I was so afraid I'd be judged as unworthy of Divine Love. But that wasn't the case. Sharing my inventory removed my distrust and opened my heart to give and receive love in a healthy way.

But taking responsibility for our part in our troubles is only another beginning. We've not yet decided whether we're ready to give up our self-defeating patterns.

Step 6. Willingness

Were entirely ready to have God remove all these defects of character.

They say at meetings that when we let go of a "defect" (what we've been calling a fearful pattern), it has scratch marks all over it. Why? Because, even though we've admitted that our old coping strategies have been blocking Love from our lives, we're not immediately willing to let go of them. Part of us still insists we need them to feel safe.

To become "entirely ready," most of us need to get so sick and tired of our old ways of handling life that we're finally willing to let them go. How wise for the founders of AA to make a space for our hesitation, to allow for patience while we wait, staying connected to our program and trusting the process.

This example illustrates how a common defect, low self-esteem, can be healed through Steps 6 and 7. My friend, DeeDee, believed the whispered lie, *They don't love me, so I must not be worthy of love.* This whispered lie and its buddy, *If they did love me, they would (or wouldn't) be doing this, saying this, etc.,* had set her up for failed relationships, addiction, codependency, and a lifetime of resentments.

As DeeDee progressed through Steps 4 and 5, she began to realize that she had set up unrealistic, unenforceable rules for how people must show her loving care. Coincidentally, she was taking a course that required her to ask her mother to list DeeDee's positive attributes. She said her mother's list felt "like a stab in the gut" because it referred to DeeDee's relapses, and implied she was better at loving her pets than her family. When DeeDee asked me for feedback, I wrote:

> "Yes. There it is in black and white. How she still judges you and withholds love. Ouch. She's right

in implying that your family relationships have been out of kilter. Alcoholism and old fears and patterns will do that. This is perfect Step-6 timing. The constant perception of 'not being lovable' has run its course and you seem 'entirely ready' to have it removed. And when you ask for its healing, your higher power will help you to see it (and your mother's reactions) differently. In the meantime, let's work on softening your heart toward your mother. Remember that she's been scared witless by your relapse earlier this year. She's human and loves you desperately while struggling to handle her fear. Here are two suggestions: Bless her by praying that she has everything that will make her happy, and then list all of her positive qualities. We'll know this pattern is healed when, regardless of what she says or does, you'll rather quickly see the love underneath her words. It may take a little time, but it will happen. Let's move on to Step 7 to get free of your old resentments."

Step 7. Humility

Humbly asked Him to remove our shortcomings.

The word *humility* is too often misunderstood as a weakness. Try thinking of it this way instead: Humility isn't thinking *less of* myself; it's thinking of myself *less often.*

In DeeDee's case, even though she had low self-esteem (thought less of herself), she spent many hours thinking of herself, rehashing how she wasn't getting loved in the ways she demanded. She couldn't humbly open her heart to her mother until she asked Loving Power to remove her resentments and self-centered demands.

The opposite of humility is false pride: *I can force the world to give me what I want.* Fortunately, we've begun to deflate our pride by admitting and listing our fears and patterns in Steps 4, 5, and 6. Now, in Step 7, we finally ask to be changed, to be free of our old heart-closing ways. Knowing we can't do it on our own, we turn to a power greater than our fears. As my friend Mark A. Lord says, "Let God (Love) do the heavy lifting." All we need to do is ask with sincerity and a willingness to get out of the way.

Here's the Seventh-Step prayer that DeeDee and I said at our next meeting.

> "My creator, I am now willing that you should have all of me, good and bad. I pray that you now remove from me every single defect of character which stands in the way of my usefulness to you and my fellows. Grant me strength as I go from here, to do your bidding."[60]

As of this writing (many months after this incident), DeeDee is open-hearted toward her mother and rarely feels rejected when her mother mentions DeeDee's past relapses. The Seventh-Step prayer worked!

Note that the Step 7 prayer asks that we be free of anything "that stands in the way of my usefulness to you [God/ Loving Energy/True Self] and my fellows." Even though we want emotional relief from our fears, problems, and isolation, our personal transformation is really about becoming useful by loving and helping others.

Step 8. Discipline

Made a list of all persons we had harmed and became willing to make amends to them all.

An amend is a mending, a closing of the separation from others. Recall the image on page 82 in Chapter 4 that showed the difference between open-hearted connection and closed-hearted separation.

We can easily discover those we have harmed by the twist of discomfort in our gut when we think of them. That discomfort is a sign of regret over our past behavior.

When listing those we've harmed, some sponsors have us make three lists: 1) *Yes, I'm willing when the time is right;* 2) *No, I'm not yet ready,* and 3) *Hell, no. Never!* The names may change lists from time to time, but for now, they just sit there. In the meantime, we trust Loving Energy and our sponsor to guide us to the right people with the right words at the right time.

Before approaching anyone to make amends, we need the discipline to reflect on our *motives*. Too often, especially early on, our motive is to get rid of our awful feelings of shame, without regard for the other person. When driven by such urges, our amends are likely to be seen as what they are: another bid to make ourselves feel better. No. This is about staying sober and loving others, unencumbered by guilt.

Again, AA's wise founders have allowed us time to become spiritually centered before we try to heal damaged relationships. In other words, we wait until we've softened our heart toward the individual. This may take a while. In my case, I had to wait five years to make amends to one of my ex-husbands. It can only happen when our hearts are ready and our motive is pure.

Step 9. Forgiveness

Made direct amends to such people wherever possible, except when to do so would injure them or others.

Forgiveness is a central piece of making amends. When our hearts are open, we can forgive the other person for their part (if any) in the incident. Then we can focus on our part and finally forgive ourselves.

Saying, "I'm sorry" is not usually sufficient, as it doesn't mend much of anything. Most people start with a statement of how much they appreciate the other person. Then they explain that they're in recovery and trying to mend their past. They briefly describe their offending words or actions, without adding the gory details. Finally, they ask the person how they can make up for the wrongdoing. If the request is possible and within reason, they do it.

Note the words at the end of Step 9: "Except when to do so would injure them or others." This means that we don't have the right to feel better at someone else's expense. Step 9 is not about blame or revenge; it's not about the past at all. It's about clearing our conscience and opening our hearts to ourselves and the other person.

Most of us fear that the person we harmed will respond with anger. Even if they do, we've learned through our step work that our security is not in someone else's hands. We've done the right thing by reaching out, and we realize the amends are about cleaning up the wreckage of our past as best we can. How the other person takes it is up to them.

Also, note the words, "made amends wherever possible." If it isn't possible, we can write a letter or imagine talking to their spirit/True Self.

Finally, let's consider the idea of *living amends*. One of the best ways to make amends with those we see often is to open our hearts to them by offering consistent kindness and compassion. We also demonstrate how we're taking good care of ourselves by conscientiously working the Steps with a sponsor. Over time, and with consistent decent behavior, we transform the damaged relationships into ones of trust and Love.

Step 10. Acceptance

Continued to take personal inventory and when we were wrong promptly admitted it.

Because we're changing a lifetime of self-centered fears and patterns, they won't all improve at once. Indeed, the more we reflect on them, the more quickly we notice when we've done or said something that doesn't align with our new, positive changes. This is where acceptance comes in. We no longer try to be perfect; we merely claim spiritual progress.

Whether the wrong is to us or another, we promptly use an abbreviated form of Steps 4–7 to look at our part. With practice, we get the hang of noticing when our old ways are disturbing our peace of mind. We do a quick personal inventory and place our fears and patterns in Love's hands. And of course, if we've harmed someone, we make amends.

Here's a rather humbling situation where an old pattern caused me to hurt another. One day at a Twelve-Step meeting, a man stood up and said very dogmatically that only the "real alcoholics" should be there. His inflexible tone sounded just like my mother when she drunkenly talked about politics, and I felt that same old fear and anger. I knew that tender spot had been triggered, but that didn't stop me from talking to him after the meeting.

Driven by my fear, I tried to convince him how his words had threatened the primary purpose of AA, to help anyone who had a desire to stop drinking. But my superior tone didn't change his mind. In fact, after a few minutes of listening to him defend his position, I grew frustrated, turned away, and said in a nasty voice, "It must be great to be so right all the time!" Oops! Self-will run riot!

Later, I did a quick inventory, admitting that I had started our conversation with a closed heart and a desire to change him, even though he'd never asked for my advice. Fear, self-deception, perfectionism, and self-condemnation had crept into my mind and closed my heart against him. After discussing the situation with my sponsor, I knew I needed to call him to confess my tender spot and apologize. Thank God, he was quite gracious about it.

That experience taught me to delay my responses when my inner child gets triggered. Instead of reacting, I need to get quiet and take good care of my own feelings. Then, and only then, if it's important to address the issue, I do. I've also learned to avoid or stay quiet around those who dogmatically insist they are right.

Step 11. Knowledge and Awareness

Sought through prayer and meditation to improve our conscious contact with God as we understood Him, praying only for knowledge of His will for us and the power to carry that out.

My AA friends say that praying is *talking to* God, and meditation is *listening* for God's response. In Chapter 3, pages 61–64, we explored meditation at length, but we haven't talked much about prayer.

Step 11 encourages us to pray "only for knowledge of His will for us and the power to carry that out." I believe that God's will is for us to open our hearts to the divine essence of every person we encounter, as stated in *ACIM* Lesson 45, "God is the mind with which I think."[61] This lesson asks me to allow Love to be the source of my thoughts. I do this by increasing my conscious contact with Loving Energy.

Early in recovery, I had never prayed and doubted that prayer would do much good. However, I decided to try it after reading Karen Casey's six persuasive reasons to pray.

1. Prayer promises relief when we are anxious.
2. Prayer connects us with our higher power when we feel isolated and full of fear.
3. Prayer frees our minds from the obsession to plan other people's lives.

4. Prayer helps us take action when we feel compelled to change the circumstances of our lives.

5. Prayer becomes a wonderful resource to draw on when living through our painful moments.

6. And prayer gives us the willingness to accept God's solution for every problem that plagues us."[62]

When I get quiet and sincerely ask to see beyond my fearful, negative thinking, I gain access to the comfort, courage, and wisdom of Loving Energy. As we commit to aligning our thoughts with Love, we will increasingly know how to handle situations that used to baffle us.

Step 12. Service and Gratitude

Having had a spiritual awakening as the result of these Steps, we tried to carry this message to alcoholics, and to practice these principles in all our affairs.

I think of a spiritual awakening as learning how to notice—and then reject—fear's destructive patterns and lies so that Loving Energy can inspire my True Self for the benefit of all.

We've heard about carrying the message to help other alcoholics, but what about practicing "these principles in all our affairs?" The short version is to strive for open-hearted living by showing Love, kindness, and care in our daily lives.

We learn to give and receive Love through relationships because we are both students and teachers to each other. Imagine several people holding hands while climbing a hill. The first person leads the person behind him, this person helps the one behind him, and so on. A stronger person helps us grow, so we can extend that strength to another. This is how recovery and most other growth paths work.

Talk to anyone who's been following a Twelve-Step program, and you'll find they've gained not only freedom from addiction, but they also enjoy loving families, amazing jobs, priceless peace of mind, and a subtle joy in life. Even when the hard times come, they have supportive love around them to help them through.

Here's a brief description of how I try to keep my recovery and spiritual growth a top priority in my life. I suggest this footwork for anyone starting any Twelve-Step recovery program.

Five Ways to Fill Up Your Serenity Bank

In early recovery, we want relief from our messy situations —right now! But rather than focusing on those situations, we need to do the necessary footwork to open our closed-off hearts to serenity and peace of mind. Think of these growth practices as ways to fill up what I call your "serenity bank." As you fill the bank through these acts of self-care, it yields miracles both inside and around you.

Five kinds of footwork fill up your serenity bank:

1. *Attend meetings:* Go early, stay late, and make sober friends (no romance!).

2. *Work the Twelve Steps with a sponsor:* Meet regularly to work on recovery.

3. *Read AA and other literature:* Fill and open your mind with wise and loving thoughts.

4. *Pray and meditate daily:* Take time to read, pray, and connect with Love.

5. *Help others (service)*: Help with group tasks, talk to newcomers, and sponsor or support others.

This table shows the difference between the alcoholic/addicted self and the sober, healthy self.

Alcoholic/Addicted Self (The Twelve Steps Reduce This)	**Sober, Healthy Self** (The Twelve Steps Increase This)
• Drugs/Alcohol, Closed Heart • Denial, Dishonesty, Criticism • Fear's Whispered Lies • "I Shall Manage" (Alcohol-ISM) • Self-Centered Fear, Self-Seeking	• Clean, Sober, Open Heart • Willingness, Honesty, Tolerance • Love's Care and Direction • God/Love's Perfect Order • Helping Others (with no strings)

Like any system, our serenity bank can get out of balance. Especially during the good times, it's easy to become complacent. Life is going so well that we forget to maintain our growth practices. At such times, our bank's riches dip dangerously low, often without our awareness. For example, we revert to old ways of "looking for love in all the wrong places," TV binging, excessive partying, seductive games, overeating, or workaholism. Perhaps we stop meeting with sober friends and start hanging out with old drinking buddies. As our serenity bank balance falls, we often find ourselves being self-centered and grouchy with our loved ones.

Fortunately, when we reach this state, we can refill our serenity bank through a crash course of footwork. We can go to extra meetings, call our sponsors, give a ride to a newcomer, or memorize a new affirmation.

When I'm running low on footwork, I often use this affirmation to flow Loving Energy into my addled mind. It opens my heart to my True Self by affirming that my troubles are simply "negative appearances" and that they can be "dissolved right now." Finally, it affirms the truth of who we are: open-hearted, loving creations. May this affirmation bless your recovery!

The Activity of God

The activity of God is the only power
At work in my mind, heart, and life.
All false beliefs, all negative appearances
Are dissolved right now
By the loving, forgiving action of God.
I am whole, strong, and free
As God created me to be.[63]

Closing Thoughts

I opened this book with a Tibetan Buddhist Prayer which expresses everything you've been reading about. If you say this prayer sincerely and regularly (as I have), and follow many of the suggestions made here, your life will be dramatically transformed.

May I be at peace, May my heart remain open.
May I awaken to the light of my own true nature.
May I be healed.
May I be a source of healing for all beings.

—Tibetan Buddhist Prayer[64]

Because we are all connected, you can say the prayer for all of us, as follows:

May we be at peace, May our hearts remain open.
May we awaken to the light of our own true nature.
May we be healed.
May we be a source of healing for all beings.

Finally, when your heart has temporarily closed against someone, you can use this prayer to reconnect your hearts.

May you be at peace, May your heart remain open.
May you awaken to the light of your own true nature.
May you be healed.
May you be a source of healing for all beings.

So, what's the payoff for all this awareness and work? I think the list of promises below describes quite well what you can expect. You won't experience each of these conditions every minute of every day. However, you will see them emerge when you continue to be honest, claim Love's power, and choose to open your heart to your True Self and the hearts of others.

Whatever growth path you're on, I'm confident that you'll be amazed by the transformation of your life. With our connected hearts, we all enjoy the following benefits.

- "We are going to know a new freedom and a new happiness.
- We will not regret the past nor wish to shut the door on it.
- We will comprehend the word *serenity* and we will know peace.
- No matter how far down the scale we have gone, we will see how our experience can benefit others.

- That feeling of uselessness and self-pity will disappear.
- We will lose interest in selfish things and gain interest in our fellows.
- Self-seeking will slip away.
- Our whole attitude and outlook upon life will change.
- Fear of people and of economic insecurity will leave us.
- We will intuitively know how to handle situations which used to baffle us.
- We will suddenly realize that God is doing for us what we could not do for ourselves."[65]

Open your heart. Open your hands. My sincere wish for you is the joyful and peaceful life that you so deserve. As we release the negative, more and more Love flows through our lives and into others, and all souls are fed!

Your Final Reflections

You might find it interesting to go back to your responses after the preface on page xxiv.

1. What has changed in how you feel about the situations that were troubling you?

2. What has helped you find greater peace of mind?
3. What new challenges have come up, and how are you attempting to switch your thoughts away from fear and negativity so you can stay positive and loving?
4. What will you do to continue your growth?
5. What benefits are you hoping for?

NOTE: In this book, I've mentioned many tools to help us open our hearts. For more specific directions for these tools, please refer to my book *50 Ways to Worry Less Now: Reject Negative Thinking to Find Peace, Clarity, and Connection.*

About the Author

Gigi Langer holds a PhD in Psychological Studies in Education and an MA in Psychology, both from Stanford University. During her twenty-five years at Eastern Michigan University, she won several awards for her teaching, and (as Georgea M. Langer) wrote four books for educators. Gigi's most recent book, *50 Ways to Worry Less Now: Reject Negative Thinking to Find Peace, Clarity, and Connection,* won a National Indie Excellence Award.

Gigi is a sought-after retreat leader and speaker who has helped thousands of people improve their lives at home and work. As a person in recovery, Gigi hasn't had a drug or drink for over thirty-five years, although she does occasionally overindulge in Ghirardelli chocolate and historical novels.

She lives happily in Florida with her husband, Peter, and her cat, Easter.

Gigi can be reached at glanger2202@gmail.com. Find her blog, newsletters, and helpful tools for recovery and personal growth at www.GigiLanger.com and most social media sites.

Notes

1 Gigi Langer, *50 Ways to Worry Less Now: Reject Negative Thinking to Find Peace, Clarity, and Connection* (Canton, MI: Possum Hill Press, 2018).

2 Shelby John, *Recovering In Recovery: The Life Changing Joy Of Sobriety* (Shelby John, 2022).

3 "Heart Disease and Mental Health Disorders," Centers for Disease Control and Prevention (CDC), reviewed May 6, 2020, https://www.cdc.gov/heartdisease/mentalhealth.htm.

4 Katherine Kam, "How Anger Can Hurt Your Heart," WebMD, reviewed on April 27, 2015, https://www.webmd.com/balance/stress-management/features/how-anger-hurts-your-heart.

5 Sonja Collins, "Work it Out: Dealing with Job Stress," WebMD, reviewed on September 12, 2012, https://www.webmd.com/mental-health/features/work-it-out-work-stress.

6 Robert A. Emmons, *Thanks!: How the New Science of Gratitude Can Make You Happier* (New York, NY: Houghton Mifflin Harcourt, 2007).

7 Amit Sood, *The Mayo Clinic Guide to Stress-Free Living* (Philadelphia, PA: Da Kapo Press, 2013).

8 Brené Brown, *The Gifts of Imperfection: Let Go of Who You Think You're Supposed to Be and Embrace Who You Are* (Center City, MN: Hazelden Publishing, 2010).

9 Gerald Jampolsky, *Love Is Letting Go of Fear* (Berkeley, CA: Celestial Arts, 1979).

10 Colin Tipping, *Radical Forgiveness: A Revolutionary Five-Stage Process to Heal Relationships, Let Go of Anger and Blame, Find Peace in Any Situation* (Louisville, CO: Sounds True, 2010).

11 Casey Klaytor, *The Light of Grace: Journeys of an Angel* (Bloomington, IN: Balboa Press, 2016).

12 Iris DeMent, "No Time To Cry" on *My Life*, Warner Brothers CD 9-45493-2, 1994, compact disc.

13 Vincent J. Felliti et al., "Relationship of Childhood Abuse and Household Dysfunction to Many of the Leading Causes of Death in Adults. The Adverse Childhood Experiences (ACE) Study," *American Journal of Preventive Medicine 14*, no. 4 (May 1998), https://doi.org/10.1016/s0749-3797(98)00017-8.

14 Elaine Aron, *The Highly Sensitive Person: How to Thrive When the World Overwhelms You* (New York: Broadway Books, 1997).

15 If your spouse or partner is accusing you of being too sensitive or insecure, please consult BrendaSchaeffer.com and her book, *Is It Love or Is It Addiction?* You may be in an unhealthy relationship.

16 Eileen Aron, Comfort Zone blog, The Highly Sensitive Person (website), accessed December 12, 2022, https://hsperson.com/comfort-zone/blog/.

17 Earnie Larsen, *Stage II Recovery: Life Beyond Addiction* (New York, NY: HarperOne, 2009).

18 Dr. Kristen Neff, "Definition of Self-Compassion," Self-Compassion.org, accessed December 12, 2022, https://self-compassion.org/the-three-elements-of-self-compassion-2/.

19 Kimberly Dawn Neumann, "What Is the Law Of Attraction?" Forbes.com, October 27, 2022, https://www.forbes.com/health/mind/what-is-law-of-attraction-loa/.

20 Jack Boland, *Master Mind Goal Achievers Journal* (Warren, MI: Master Mind Publishing Company, 1992).

21 "Lesson 188," A Course in Miracles, acim.org, 2007, https://acim.org/acim/lesson-188/the-peace-of-god-is-shining-in-me-now/en/s/596.

22 Anonymous, "Your open talk," email to Gigi Langer, November 20, 2019.

23 Ram Dass, *Be Here Now* (New York, NY: Harper One, 2010).

24 Kendra Cherry, "What is Mindfulness Meditation?" VeryWellMind, updated September 22, 2022, https://www.verywellmind.com/mindfulness-meditation-88369.

25 "21-Day Meditation Challenge," deepakchopra.com, April 21, 2022, https://www.deepakchopra.com/articles/21-day-meditation-challenge/.

26 Deepak Chopra, "21-Day Meditation Experience—Energy of Attraction CDs," October 29, 2014, https://www.amazon.com/dp/B00OZY51TW.

27 Susan Morales, "How Not to Meditate," email to Gigi Langer, November 10, 2017.

28 Cherry, "What is Mindfulness Meditation?"

29 Melody Beatty, "Letting Go of Urgency," *The Language of Letting Go: Daily Meditations for Codependents* (Center City, MN: Hazelden Publishing, 1990).

30 Beth Ann Mayer, "How to Use Mindfulness-Based Stress Reduction for Mental Well Being," HealthLine.com, February 2022, https://www.healthline.com/health/mindfulness-based-stress-reduction#what-it-is.

31 Laura Madson et al., "Effectiveness of mindfulness-based stress reduction in a self-selecting and self-paying community setting," *Clinical Psychiatry 30*, no. 1 (2018):52–60.

32 Muriel Barbery, *The Elegance of the Hedgehog*, trans. by Alison Anderson (New York, NY: Europa Editions, 2008).

33 Joe Dispenza, *Evolve Your Brain: The Science of Changing Your Mind* (Deerfield Beach, FL: Health Communications, Inc., 2008); Rick Hansen and Richard Mendius, *Buddha's Brain: The Practical Neuroscience of Happiness, Love, and Wisdom* (New York, NY: New Harbinger, 2009).

34 Andrew Lloyd Weber and Tim Rice, "Everything's Alright," *Jesus Christ Superstar*, October 16, 1970.

35 Kam, "How Anger Can Hurt Your Heart."

36 Rumi as quoted by Timothy Freke, *Rumi Wisdom: Daily Teachings from the Great Sufi Master* (New York, NY: Sterling, 2003).

37 The four "barriers to Love" are derived from *Alcoholics Anonymous*, page 84–86 (resentment, selfishness, dishonesty, or fear). I didn't list "fear" separately, as it underlies each barrier. I added the last item, Self-Condemnation, as it's a common fear-driven barrier.

38 EMDR facilitates the accessing and processing of traumatic memories and other adverse life experiences to relieve affective distress, reformulate negative beliefs, and reduce physiological arousal.

39 Gerald Jampolsky, *Teach Only Love: The Twelve Principles of Attitudinal Healing* (Hillsboro, OR: Beyond Words Publishing, 2000).

40 Freddie van Rensburg, *Life Anon: A Twelve-Step Guide to Life* (Freddie van Rensburg, 2019).

41 Don Miguel Ruiz and Janet Mills, *The Four Agreements: A Practical Guide to Personal Freedom* (San Rafael, CA: Amber-Allen Publishing, 2011).

42 Eckhardt Tolle, The Power of Now: *A Guide to Spiritual Enlightenment* (Novato, CA: New World Library, 1997).

43 Pema Chödrön, *When Things Fall Apart: Heart Advice for Difficult Times* (Boulder, CO: Shambhala, 2016).

44 Mayer, "How to Use Mindfulness-Based Stress Reduction for Mental Well Being."

45 "Lesson 204," A Course in Miracles, acim.org, accessed December 12, 2022.

46 Byron Katie. *Loving What Is: Four Questions That Can Change Your Life* (New York, NY: Three Rivers Press, 2003).

47 Steven Pressfield, *The War of Art. Winning the Inner Creative Battle* (New York, NY: Warner Books, 2003).

48 Karen Casey, *Daily Meditations for Practicing The Course* (Center City, MN: Hazelden, 1995).

49 Richard Rohr, "Some Simple But Urgent Guidance to Get Us Through These Next Few Months," personal email, September 19, 2020.

50 Alcoholics Anonymous, *Alcoholics Anonymous: The Story of How Many Thousands of Men and Women Have Recovered from Alcoholism* (New York, NY: Alcoholics Anonymous World Services, 2002), 66.

51 Buddy T , "Recognizing alcoholism as a disease," VeryWellMind, updated March 17, 2021, https://www.verywellmind.com/alcoholism-as-a-disease-63292.

52 Markus Heilig et al., "Addiction as a brain disease revised: why it still matters, and the need for consilience," *Neuropsychopharmacology 46*, no. 10 (September 2021): 1715–1723.

53 Marissa B. Esser et al., "Deaths and Years of Potential Life Lost From Excessive Alcohol Use—United States, 2011–2015," *MMWR Morb Mortal Wkly Rep* 69 (2020):1428–1433, http://dx.doi.org/10.15585/mmwr.mm6939a6externalicon.

54 Esser, "Deaths and Years."

55 Psychology Today Staff, "What Is Addiction?" PsychologyToday.com, accessed December 13, 2022, https://www.psychologytoday.com/us/basics/addiction.

56 Mandy Erickson, "Alcoholics Anonymous most effective path to alcohol abstinence," Stanford Medicine News, March 11, 2020, https://med.stanford.edu/news/all-news/2020/03/alcoholics-anonymous-most-effective-path-to-alcohol-abstinence.html.

57 Erickson, "Alcoholics Anonymous most effective path."

58 Erickson, "Alcoholics Anonymous most effective path."

59 Alcoholics Anonymous, *Alcoholics Anonymous: The Story of How Many Thousands of Men and Women Have Recovered from Alcoholism* (New York, NY: Alcoholics Anonymous World Services, 2002), 63.

60 Alcoholics Anonymous, *Alcoholics Anonymous: The Story of How Many Thousands of Men and Women Have Recovered from Alcoholism* (New York, NY: Alcoholics Anonymous World Services, 2002), 76.

61 "Lesson 45," A Course in Miracles, acim.org, accessed December 13, 2022.

62 Karen Casey, *A Life of My Own: Meditations on Hope and Acceptance* (Center City, MN: Hazelden Publishing, 1993).

63 J. Sig Paulson, "The Activity of God," *Walking with God* (pamphlet) (Unity Village, MO: Unity School of Christianity, 1970).

64 "Tibetan Buddhist Prayer," Unitarian Universalist Association, uua.org, accessed December 13, 2022, https://www.uua.org/worship/words/prayer/tibetan-buddhist-prayer.

65 Alcoholics Anonymous, *Alcoholics Anonymous: The Story of How Many Thousands of Men and Women Have Recovered from Alcoholism* (New York, NY: Alcoholics Anonymous World Services, 2002), 83–84.

www.ingramcontent.com/pod-product-compliance
Lightning Source LLC
Chambersburg PA
CBHW060951050426
42337CB00054B/3905
9780999122051